EVIDENCE-BASED DECISION MAKING

A TRANSLATIONAL GUIDE
FOR DENTAL PROFESSIONALS

EVIDENCE-BASED DECISION MAKING

A TRANSLATIONAL GUIDE
FOR DENTAL PROFESSIONALS

Jane L. Forrest, EdD, RDH

Chair, Health Promotion, Disease Prevention, and Epidemiology
University of Southern California School of Dentistry
Los Angeles, CA

Syrene A. Miller, BA

Project Manager
National Center for Dental Hygiene Research
Colbert, WA

Pam R. Overman, BSDH, EdD

Associate Dean for Academic Affairs
University of Missouri-Kansas City School of Dentistry
Kansas City, MO

Michael G. Newman, DDS

Adjunct Professor Emeritus
Editor and Chief, Journal of Evidence-Based Dental Practice
UCLA School of Dentistry
Los Angeles, CA

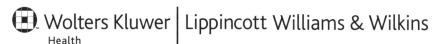

Wolters Kluwer | Lippincott Williams & Wilkins
Health

Philadelphia • Baltimore • New York • London
Buenos Aires • Hong Kong • Sydney • Tokyo

Acquisitions Editor: Barrett Koger
Managing Editor: Andrea M. Klingler
Marketing Manager: Nancy Bradshaw
Production Editor: John Larkin
Designer: Stephen Druding
Compositor: Aptara, Inc.

First Edition

Library of Congress Cataloging-in-Publication Data

Evidence-based decision making : a translational guide for dental professionals / Jane L.
    Forrest . . . [et al.] —1st ed.
        p. ; cm.
    Includes bibliographical references and index.
    ISBN-13: 978-0-7817-6533-6
    ISBN-10: 0-7817-6533-1
    1. Evidence-based dentistry.   2. Dentistry—Decision making   I. Forrest, Jane L.
    [DNLM: 1. Decision Support Techniques.   2. Dental Care.   3. Evidence-Based Medicine.
    4. Practice Management, Dental.   WU 29 E928 2008]
    RK51.5.E95 2008
    617.6—dc22

                                                                    2008010762

Care has been taken to confirm the accuracy of the information present and to describe generally accepted practices. However, the authors, editors, and publisher are not responsible for errors or omissions or for any consequences from application of the information in this book and make no warranty, expressed or implied, with respect to the currency, completeness, or accuracy of the contents of the publication. Application of this information in a particular situation remains the professional responsibility of the practitioner; the clinical treatments described and recommended may not be considered absolute and universal recommendations.

The authors, editors, and publisher have exerted every effort to ensure that drug selection and dosage set forth in this text are in accordance with the current recommendations and practice at the time of publication. However, in view of ongoing research, changes in government regulations, and the constant flow of information relating to drug therapy and drug reactions, the reader is urged to check the package insert for each drug for any change in indications and dosage and for added warnings and precautions. This is particularly important when the recommended agent is a new or infrequently employed drug.

Some drugs and medical devices presented in this publication have Food and Drug Administration (FDA) clearance for limited use in restricted research settings. It is the responsibility of the health care provider to ascertain the FDA status of each drug or device planned for use in their clinical practice.

To purchase additional copies of this book, call our customer service department at **(800) 638-3030** or fax orders to **(301) 223-2320**. International customers should call **(301) 223-2300**.

Visit Lippincott Williams & Wilkins on the Internet: http://www.lww.com. Lippincott Williams & Wilkins customer service representatives are available from 8:30 am to 6:00 pm, EST.

To our family and friends, whose love and support make all things possible.

PREFACE

Evidence-based decision making (EBDM) is the formalized process of using a specific set of skills for identifying, searching for, and interpreting clinical and scientific evidence so that it can be used at the point of care. The evidence is considered in conjunction with the clinician's experience and judgment, the patient's preferences and values, and the clinical/patient circumstances. *Evidence-Based Decision Making: A Translational Guide for Dental Professionals* teaches the skills necessary for lifelong learning that are an important part of the ability to translate recent and relevant scientific evidence into practical applications.

EBDM is an essential tool that is used to improve the quality of care and to reduce the gap between what we know, what is possible, and what we do. An evidence-based health care decision is one that includes the decision maker's ability to find, assess, and incorporate high-quality valid information in the process. New electronic products, systems, and resources associated with clinical decision support also will require the end user to be competent in EBDM.

ORGANIZATION

This book presents content centered on the essential and fundamental skills of EBDM. *Evidence-Based Decision Making: A Translational Guide for Dental Professionals* provides succinct information in nine chapters, beginning in Chapter 1 with an introduction to EBDM concepts and the five essential skills. Chapters 2 through 4 focus on *Skill 1. Converting Information Needs/Problems into Clinical Questions So That They Can Be Answered.* In these chapters, the reader will learn how to formulate background and foreground (PICO) questions, identify the type of question being asked, and select the appropriate type of studies related to the question, as well as how the levels of evidence relate to specific types of studies. Chapter 5 reviews *Skill 2. Conducting a Computerized Search with Maximum Efficiency for Finding the Best External Evidence with Which to Answer the Question.* Readers will learn how the PICO question relates to identifying key terms and developing an efficient search strategy to find relevant evidence. Chapters 6 and 7 focus on *Skill 3. Critically Appraising the Evidence for Its Validity and Usefulness* and teach the reader how to critically appraise relevant evidence, evaluate Internet Web sites, and summarize the results. Chapter 8 covers *Skill 4. Applying the Results of the Appraisal, or Evidence, in*

Clinical Practice. Readers will learn how to use critical thinking to apply the evidence. This incorporates the use of patient care outcome measures and the consideration of the patients' circumstances, preferences, or values, along with the clinician's experience and judgment and the scientific evidence to formulate the final decision with the patient. The book concludes with Chapter 9, which discusses *Skill 5. Evaluating the Process and Your Performance.* This brings the EBDM process full circle, allowing readers to conduct a self-evaluation of each aspect of the process and outlining how to strengthen their EBDM skills.

FEATURES

An algorithm displaying the EBDM process and skills is included at the beginning of each chapter, allowing the reader to understand the progression involved in learning the EBDM process and the focus of that particular chapter of the book. To facilitate learning, each chapter of *Evidence-Based Decision Making: A Translational Guide for Dental Professionals* has specific **Objectives** and contains **Suggested Activities: a Quiz, Critical Thinking Questions,** and **Exercises,** all of which are meant to reinforce learning and encourage discussion. The Quizzes and Critical Thinking Questions are specifically developed to strengthen the reader's understanding of concepts. The Exercises are designed to take the reader through the skill development process necessary to use EBDM. A consistent patient case is used throughout the book to model and teach the concepts in each chapter. Five **Case Scenarios** are used in the exercises and are meant to give the reader more opportunities to apply EBDM skills as they progress.

When readers are finished with *Evidence-Based Decision Making: A Translational Guide for Dental Professionals*, it is expected that they will have completed the entire process for each type of clinical question that arises in practice: therapy/prevention, diagnosis, etiology/harm/causation, and prognosis. By completing all steps for each case, an EBDM portfolio can be created that can be used as a guide for future reference.

This book reflects many years of cumulative experience in designing educational materials, facilitating workshops, editing journals, and educating health professionals about how to integrate the evidence-based process into practice. The easy-to-read content and highly instructional exercises will be helpful as you progress through the EBDM process. Mastering these skills will foster better communication with colleagues and patients, which will ultimately result in better health care for our patients.

ADDITIONAL RESOURCES

Evidence-Based Decision Making: A Translational Guide for Dental Professionals includes additional resources for both instructors and students that are available on the book's companion Web site at thepoint.lww.com/forrest.

Instructors

Approved adopting instructors will be given access to an Instructor's Manual that includes the following additional resources:

* PowerPoint presentations
* Quizzes and Quiz Answer Keys
* Exercises and Critical Thinking Activities
* Suggested Activities
* WebCT and Blackboard-Ready Cartridges

Students

Students who have purchased *Evidence-Based Decision Making: A Translational Guide for Dental Professionals* have access to the following additional resources:

* Quizzes
* Exercises and Critical Thinking Activities

Jane L. Forrest
Syrene A. Miller
Pamela R. Overman
Michael G. Newman

CONTENTS

CHAPTER 1

Introduction to Evidence-Based Decision Making

PURPOSE

The purpose of this section is to introduce basic concepts and define evidence-based decision making (EBDM).

OBJECTIVES

After completing this chapter, the reader will be able to:

1. Discuss the evolution of the evidence-based approach, and describe how it influences the education and practice of dentistry and dental hygiene today.
2. Define EBDM and discuss its purpose.
3. Identify and discuss the four primary reasons EBDM is critical for health care providers.
4. Describe the five steps and skills necessary to perform EBDM.
5. Explain the benefits of EBDM.
6. Discuss at least one research study that supports the integration of EBDM into clinical practice.

SUGGESTED ACTIVITIES

Quiz
Critical Thinking Questions
Exercise 1-1

EVOLUTION OF THE EVIDENCE-BASED APPROACH

The evidence-based process was introduced at McMaster University, Ontario, Canada, in the 1980s to overcome many of the deficiencies of traditional experienced-based education and in response to the need to improve the quality of health care by closing the gap between what is known (research) and what is practiced.[1-4] The term *evidence-based medicine* (EBM) was first used to describe a method of mastering self-directed, lifelong learning skills and a new paradigm for medical practice[5] and is defined as "the integration of best research evidence with clinical expertise and patient values."[6] At McMaster, this method incorporated the faculty's use of problem-based learning and their development of a systematic approach to using evidence to answer questions and direct clinical action. The early developers of EBM realized how medical practice was changing with the increase in clinical research and the need to use the medical literature to guide practice. The randomized clinical trial (RCT) had become the standard for demonstrating efficacy for drugs, surgical procedures, and diagnostic tests.[5]

PURPOSE AND DEFINITION OF EVIDENCE-BASED DECISION MAKING

As EBM has evolved, so has the realization that the evidence from scientific research is only one key component of the decision-making process and does not tell a practitioner what to do. The use of current best evidence does *not* replace clinical expertise or input from the patient, but rather provides another dimension to the decision-making process that is also placed in context with the patient's clinical circumstances (Fig. 1–1). It is this decision-making process that is termed *evidence-based decision making* (EBDM) and is defined as the formalized process of using the skills for identifying, searching for, and interpreting the results of the best scientific evidence, which is considered in conjunction with the clinician's experience and judgment, the patient's preferences and values, and the clinical/patient circumstances when making patient care decisions. EBDM is not unique to medicine or any specific health discipline, but represents a concise way of referring to the application of evidence to the decision-making process.

EBDM is about solving clinical problems and involves two fundamental principles: evidence alone is never sufficient to make a clinical decision, and a hierarchy of evidence exists to guide clinical decision making.[7,8] EBDM recognizes that clinicians can never have complete knowledge about all conditions, medications, materials, or available products and provides a mechanism for assimilating current research findings into everyday practice to provide the best possible patient care.

THE NEED FOR EVIDENCE-BASED DECISION MAKING

Forces driving the need for EBDM to improve the quality of care are: variations in practice; slow translation and

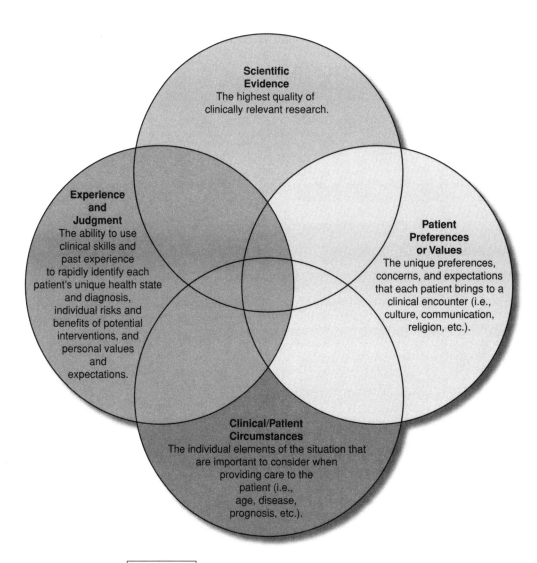

Scientific Evidence
The highest quality of clinically relevant research.

Experience and Judgment
The ability to use clinical skills and past experience to rapidly identify each patient's unique health state and diagnosis, individual risks and benefits of potential interventions, and personal values and expectations.

Patient Preferences or Values
The unique preferences, concerns, and expectations that each patient brings to a clinical encounter (i.e., culture, communication, religion, etc.).

Clinical/Patient Circumstances
The individual elements of the situation that are important to consider when providing care to the patient (i.e., age, disease, prognosis, etc.).

FIGURE 1–1 Evidence-based decision making process.

assimilation of the scientific evidence into practice;[1-3,9] managing the information overload; and changing educational competencies that require students to have the skills for lifelong learning.[10]

Variations in Practice Patterns

Substantial advances have been made in our knowledge of effective disease prevention measures and of new therapies, diagnostic tests, materials, techniques, and delivery systems, and yet the translation of this knowledge into practice has not been fully applied. Variations in practices among dental and dental hygiene clinicians are well documented, whether it involves diagnostic procedures, treatment planning,[11,12] or prescribing antibiotics.[13,14] In addition, other factors contributing to variations in practice are the inconsistencies among schools in what is taught and emphasized and the expectations and procedures tested by state and regional dental licensing boards.

Slow Translation and Assimilation of Research Findings into Practice

Far too often, variations in practice occur from a gap between the time current research knowledge becomes available and its application to care. Consequently, there is a delay in adopting useful procedures and in discontinuing ineffective or harmful ones.[15-18] Assimilating scientific evidence into practice requires that clinicians keep up to date by reading extensively, attending courses, and taking advantage of the Internet and electronic databases to search for published scientific articles. However, colleagues and personal journal collections continue to be the dominant information sources for treatment decisions, rather than using electronic databases to access the most current scientific literature.[19-22] Treatment decisions also tend to reflect the knowledge, skills, and attitudes learned as a student,[18,23-25] and trends indicating that the longer clinicians are out of school, the bigger the gap in their knowledge of up-to-date care.[8,23,24,26,27] This reinforces the need to learn evidence-based information seeking behaviors and critical analysis skills while still in school.

Managing the Information Overload

In addition to influencing variations in practice and the slow translation and assimilation of scientific evidence into practice, the rate at which information is increasing is greater than any one person can possibly read and remember. With the number of good clinical trials and meta-analyses increasing at a rate of 10% per year[27] and located in more than 700 dental journals worldwide, knowing which journals to subscribe to that are related to an individual's practice is nearly impossible. Niederman found that in order to keep up to date with just the RCTs addressing therapy, one would have to read six articles per week, 52 weeks per year.[27] This number increases as articles related to diagnosis, prognosis, etiology, or harm are considered.

Forrest and Miller[28] found a substantial number of articles, 112 meta-analyses (reviews and statistical analysis of already conducted research that address the same question) and 1,700 RCTs, published between 1990 and 2003 when searching MEDLINE for evidence that supports clinical dental hygiene practice. In this case, 50% of the 112 meta-analyses were located in seven journals (*British Dental Journal, Caries Research, Community Dentistry & Oral Epidemiology, Journal of the ADA, Journal of Clinical Dentistry, Journal of Clinical Periodontology,* and the *Journal of Public Health Dentistry*) and the Cochrane Library with the remaining half found in 33 other journals. Of the 1,700 RCTs, 70% were located in 32 journals with the remaining 30% in 174 journals.[28]

The challenge is to find relevant clinical evidence when it's needed to help make well-informed decisions. The EBDM process provides us with an approach to answer this challenge. Evidence-based practice is now possible because of increased access to relevant clinical findings via development of online databases and computers that enable quick access to the scientific literature. Being able to search electronically across hundreds of journals for specific answers to patient questions or problems solves this problem.

Not only is access available for practitioners, but many of the same resources are available to the general public. Consumers are learning about research designs and levels of evidence as more health-related information gains popular attention.[28-31] The EBDM process becomes more critical as patients become more informed health care consumers. Patients increasingly use the Internet as a resource for information about health care options and procedures. As early as the year 2000, 93 million Americans were using the Internet to research at least one of 16 major health topics and 77 million American adults said they went online to look for health or medical information.[32]

Patients come to their appointments educated (sometimes inaccurately) about new dental products, treatment procedures, and diagnostic tests they have learned about through advertisements and the Internet. However, many of the resources available to the general public are biased, inaccurate, or not appropriate for the patient. It is important for practitioners to develop the skills to analyze and evaluate these sources to accurately address patients' concerns with valid evidence. The ability to do this while integrating good science with clinical judgment enhances credibility, builds trust and confidence with the patient, and may enhance the patient's quality of care. Table 1–1 highlights the first three forces driving the need for EBDM.

Changing Educational Requirements

Another need for EBDM is reflected in educational requirements and competencies. Traditional health professional curricula have been directed toward memorizing facts in a dense-packed format with insufficient time for reflection and little or no self-directed learning.[34] In dental and dental hygiene education, a focus on technical skills, coupled with a division of preclinical/clinical course material, has historically delayed clinical experiences. Integration of the basic sciences with preclinical work and patient care is often lacking, resulting in a gap between learning technical skills and clinical reasoning. The preclinical training approach, in effect, postpones the development of clinical judgment and linkage of the biomedical sciences to clinical reasoning and patient care. Traditional curricula also create a dependency on faculty to teach students rather than on facilitating the students' assumption of responsibility for their own learning.[34]

Besides the need for redefined clinical skills, virtually all reports addressing curriculum reform in health professional education identify information management, technology, high-level thinking, and problem-solving skills as needed competencies.[10,35] Growth in professional literature, pressure from economic forces, and availability of newer information technology reinforce the need for professionals to develop information management skills, which are emphasized in an evidence-based curriculum. A comparison of traditional and EB curricula is presented in Table 1–2.

EBDM SKILLS AND THE FIVE-STEP PROCESS

The principles of EBDM methodology are based on the abilities to critically appraise and correctly apply

TABLE 1-1

The Need for Evidence-Based Decision-Making Process (EBDM)

Forces Driving the Need	Problem	Result of Using EBDM
Variations in practice	Translation of research for use in practice is not fully applied so that patients receive the best possible care	Enhances consistency of practice Increases standards of practice and practice guidelines based on scientific evidence
Slow translation and assimilation of research into practice	Patients do not receive the best possible care as soon as it is available and ineffective care is not discontinued	Allows clinicians to stay current to close the gap between what is known and what is practiced
Managing the information overload	Ability to keep up with the increasing publication of clinical research studies in multiple journals and databases. Also, quick access to health information and new products and procedures is now available; however, not all sources are accurate and can be misleading or inappropriate	Access to computers and online databases (e.g., PubMed) allow clinicians to quickly find research evidence to accurately answer questions and provide patient-centered care that is based on an evaluation of the most recent scientific findings

current evidence from relevant research to decisions made in practice so that what is known is reflected in the care provided. EBDM includes the process of systematically finding, appraising, and using current research findings in making clinical decisions. EBDM requires understanding new concepts and developing new skills, such as asking good clinical questions, conducting an efficient computerized search, critically appraising the evidence, applying the results in clinical practice, and evaluating the outcomes. The five-step process is outlined in Table 1–3. Figure 1–2 displays the algorithm for the EBDM process.

Understanding the basic concepts used in EBDM builds the foundation for developing the necessary skills needed to use the process. The following procedures provide an overview of the five steps and skills involved in establishing an evidence-based practice.

Converting Information Needs/Problems into Clinical Questions so that they can be Answered

The evidence-based approach guides clinicians in structuring well-built questions that result in patient-centered answers that can improve the quality of care and patient satisfaction. Asking the right question is a difficult skill to learn, yet it is fundamental to evidence-based practice. The process almost always begins with a patient question or problem. A "well-built" question should include four parts, referred to as PICO, that identify the patient problem or population (P), intervention (I), comparison

TABLE 1-2

Traditional vs. Evidence-Based Curricula

Traditional Curricula	Evidence-Based Curricula
Directed toward memorizing facts	Provides a formalized structure for integrating evidence into decisions made about patient care
Insufficient time for reflection	Incorporates time for students to find answers to their questions
Little or no self-directed learning	Self-directed
Focus on technical skills Division of preclinical/clinical course material	Integrates the need for scientific evidence in relation to patient care/circumstances
Dependency on faculty to teach students	Requires students to access the scientific evidence to answer clinical questions and develops the skills for life-long learning

TABLE 1-3

Skills Needed to Apply the Evidence-Based Decision-Making Process[8]

- Convert information needs/problems into clinical questions so that they can be answered
- Conduct a computerized search with maximum efficiency for finding the best external evidence with which to answer the question
- Critically appraise the evidence for its validity and usefulness (clinical applicability)
- Apply the results of the appraisal, or evidence, in clinical practice
- Evaluate the process and your performance

(C), and outcome(s) (O).[8] This will be discussed in more depth in the following section.

Conducting a Computerized Search with Maximum Efficiency for Finding the Best External Evidence with which to Answer the Question

Finding relevant evidence requires conducting a focused search of the peer-reviewed professional literature based on the appropriate methodology. An understanding of how to use the terminology, filters, and features of the biomedical databases maximizes the effectiveness of the literature search. Chapter 5 will detail this process more fully.

Critically Appraising the Evidence for its Validity and Usefulness (Clinical Applicability)

After you have found the most current evidence, the next step in the EBDM process is to understand what you have and its relevance to your patient and PICO question. Knowing what constitutes the highest levels of evidence and having a basic understanding of research design are the foundation of acquiring the skills to appraise the scientific literature to answer questions and keep current with practice. Worksheets are available to guide the critical appraisal process through prompts that aid in determining the strengths, weaknesses, and validity of a study. This will be discussed more fully in Chapter 6 and Chapter 7.

Applying the Results of the Appraisal, or Evidence, in Clinical Practice

A key component of the fourth step is determining whether the findings are relevant to the patient, problem, or question. Presenting information to patients in a clear and unambiguous manner will help translate research into practice. This skill will be outlined in Chapter 8.

Evaluating the Process and Your Performance

After making a decision and implementing a course of treatment, evaluating the outcomes is the final step. Evaluating the process may include a range of activities such as examining outcomes related to the health/function of the patient, patient satisfaction and input into the decision-making process, and a self-evaluation of how well each step of the EBDM process was conducted. With an understanding of how to effectively use EBDM, one can quickly and conveniently stay current with scientific findings on topics that are important. Chapter 9 will cover this topic.

THE EVIDENCE FOR EVIDENCE-BASED DECISION MAKING

There is a growing body of research related to implementing EBDM into curricula for predoctoral students and postgraduate residents. Consistent themes have emerged identifying characteristics of programs that are effective in changing knowledge using the scientific literature and critical appraisal skills; however, most of these studies provide weak evidence in that none have looked at long-term behaviors that ultimately benefit patient outcomes. Findings from systematic reviews (that is, reviews of already conducted research that address the same question), RCTs, and qualitative studies that addressed predoctoral and postgraduate medical, dental, and dental hygiene education were reviewed to substantiate the benefits of using and incorporating EBDM into education.[36,37]

The objective of an SR, *Implementing Evidence-Based Practice in Undergraduate Teaching Clinics: A Systematic Review and Recommendations*,[38] was to identify effective strategies for promoting and implementing EBDM clinical practice in undergraduate dental education.[38] Twelve studies met the inclusion criteria, including nine original research studies and three SRs. Of the nine original research studies, only three examined the application of EBDM skills in real-time patient situations. The first study evaluated a focused educational intervention on the use of MEDLINE and critical appraisal skills in undergraduate medical education.[39] During a 4-week course, students developed and applied EB skills (e.g., formulating focused clinical questions from patient care problems encountered in their clinical rotation, conducting an efficient MEDLINE search, critically appraising retrieved articles, and applying the evidence to the patient problem).

Pre- and post-assessments were conducted of students' reading/library behaviors, skills, and attitudes on issues relating to EBDM. Significant differences were found between intervention and control groups in self-assessed MEDLINE and critical appraisal

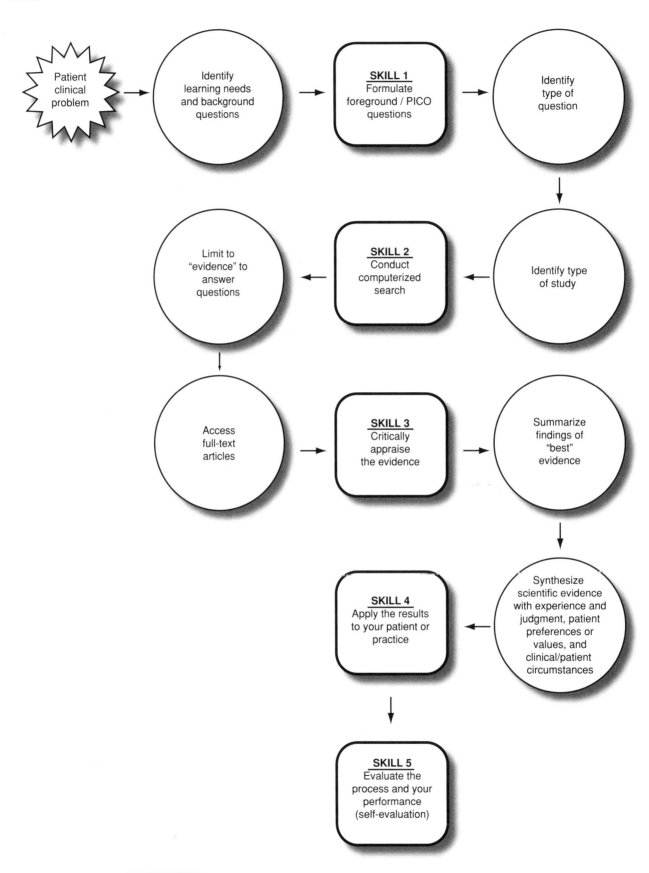

FIGURE 1–2   The algorithm for the evidence-based decision-making process

skills—$p < 0.002$ and $p < 0.0002$, respectively.[39] Although enhanced skills at retrieving journal articles were not statistically significant, the tendency to use original research articles to answer patient care questions was statistically higher in the intervention group, $p < 0.0008$. Success of the course was credited to the active involvement of faculty and students, the clinical relevance of learning exercises, and the integration of all EBDM skills into clinical practice.[39] These findings were similar to the other studies where active learning strategies were used and there was continuity between theory and application to patient care.[40]

In summary,

1. Findings reinforce the need to integrate EBDM into routine clinical practice to affect positive changes in knowledge, critical appraisal skills, attitudes, and behavior, which ultimately may benefit patient care.
2. Teaching should take place in "real time" versus in a standalone course so that both EBM skills and application of the best available evidence is used in direct patient care building on what might have been taught in a classroom case or simulation.[41]

EDUCATIONAL STANDARDS FOR EVIDENCE-BASED DENTISTRY AND DENTAL HYGIENE

Since the 1990s, the evidence-based "movement" has continued to advance and is becoming widely accepted among the health care professions, with many adopting its principles and incorporating them into specific competencies for education. For example, the American Dental Association has defined evidence-based dentistry as follows:[42]

> Evidence-based dentistry (EBD) is an approach to oral health care that requires the judicious integration of systematic assessments of clinically relevant scientific evidence, relating to the patient's oral and medical condition and history, with the dentist's clinical expertise and the patient's treatment needs and preferences.

The ADA Accreditation Standards for Dental Education Programs now expect dental schools to develop specific competencies that are reflective of an evidence-based definition of general dentistry, which

> ...means that the dentist integrates individual clinical expertise with the best available external clinical evidence from systematic clinical research. Individual clinical expertise includes effective and efficient diagnosis and thoughtful identification and compassionate use of individual patients' predicaments, rights and preferences in making clinical decisions about care (p. 7).[43]

Core Competencies

Core competencies, identified by the American Dental Education Association (ADEA), focus on the need for graduates to become critical thinkers, problem solvers, and consumers of current research findings to the point that they become lifelong learners. These skills parallel those of evidence-based practice by teaching students to find, evaluate, and incorporate current evidence into their decision making.[44,45]

Competencies for dental hygienists are incorporated in the ADEA Dental Hygiene Curriculum Guidelines.[46] For example, under Clinical Dental Hygiene, I. Introduction, Definitions, Process of Care (p. 10), is the statement: "The process of care requires defined problem solving and critical thinking skills and supports evidenced-based decision-making." A similar statement is found under the Community Dental Health for Dental Hygienists section related to research in that students are expected to learn basic principles of research methodology and biostatistics, including application of this knowledge to evaluate literature provided by various sources and apply it to evidenced-based dental hygiene practice (p. 14). Further support for EBDM is found in the curriculum guidelines under Research for Dental and Dental Hygiene Education (pp. 123–128)[46] in that their aims are to provide both dentists and dental hygienists with the skills and knowledge to be able to access the most recent and relevant scientific evidence, critically appraise it, and determine if it is applicable to the problem being addressed. The clear and unambiguous intent of the accreditation standards and competencies contained within the ADA and ADEA documents are the importance of comprehensive patient-centered care and the need for adding EBDM to the traditional experienced-based decision-making approach. These are summarized in Table 1–4.

EVIDENCE-BASED DECISION MAKING IN CLINICAL PRACTICE

The dentists in a state-of-the-art practice in Deer Park, Washington, are using EBDM. When questions arise from patients or staff, the dentists and hygienists incorporate current scientific evidence in the decision-making process. For example, when a hygienist questioned why the office used a specific type of dental floss and suggested that another floss was more effective in preventing interproximal caries, the dentists turned to the current scientific literature and presented the findings to the hygienist and other office staff for discussion.[47] In another case, a patient presented with burning mouth syndrome and again the dentists turned to the scientific literature. They used the EBDM process to find evidence on the options to relieve the symptoms of burning mouth syndrome.[48] Recently, a patient with severe periodontal disease

TABLE 1-4

Educational Competencies for Evidence-Based Decision-Making Process in Dentistry and Dental Hygiene

American Dental Association Competencies		*American Dental Education Association Competencies*	
Dentistry	*Dental Hygiene*	*Dentistry*	*Dental Hygiene*
Standard 2 *Biomedical Sciences, 2-15:* Biomedical science knowledge *must* be of sufficient depth and scope for graduates to apply advances in modern biology to clinical practice and to integrate new medical knowledge and therapies relevant to oral health care. *Ethics and Professionalism, 2-22:* Graduates *must* recognize the role of lifelong learning and self-assessment in maintaining competency. *Information Management and Critical Thinking 2-23:* Graduates *must* be competent in the use of critical thinking and problem solving related to the comprehensive care of patients. *2-24:* Graduates *must* be competent in the use of information technology resources in contemporary dental practice.	*ADA 2-25:* Graduates must be competent in the application of self-assessment skills to prepare them for lifelong learning. The intent is that dental hygienists should possess self-assessment skills as a foundation for maintaining competency and quality assurance. *ADA 2-26:* Graduates must be competent in the evaluation of current scientific literature. The intent is that dental hygienists should have the ability to evaluate scientific literature as a foundation for lifelong learning and adapting to changes in healthcare. *ADA 2-27:* Graduates must be competent in problem solving strategies related to comprehensive patient care and management of patients. The intent is that critical thinking and decision making skills are necessary to provide effective and efficient dental hygiene services.	Continuously analyze the outcomes of patient treatment to improve that treatment. Evaluate scientific literature and other sources of information to make decisions about dental treatment. Manage oral health based on an application of scientific principles.	*11.* Evaluate published clinical and basic science research and integrate this information to improve the oral health of the patient. *13.* Accept responsibility for solving problems and making decisions based on accepted scientific principles.

questioned if hormone replacement therapy would decrease her bone loss. Again, the dentists in Deer Park used the EBDM process to answer the patient's question.

CONCLUSION

Through this approach, there is an understanding of how the literature should be appraised and what constitutes good evidence. Using this foundation of EBDM helps assure that practices are clinically sound and focused on the best possible outcomes. Evidence-based practice also contributes to continuously improving effectiveness, appropriateness, and quality of care. This allows practices to be consistent with risk management principles and easily substantiate the care provided to patients, policy makers, and insurance companies.

An EBDM approach closes the gap between clinical research and the realities of practice by providing dental practitioners with the skills to find, efficiently filter, interpret, and apply research findings so that what is known is reflected in what we do. This approach assists clinicians in keeping current with conditions a patient may have by providing a mechanism for addressing gaps in knowledge and provide the best care possible. For an EBDM approach to become the norm for practice, it must be integrated throughout educational programs and used in developing sound clinical guidelines. It is important that faculty members have the EBDM skills expected of their students and create an environment in which students become self-directed learners. Students and practitioners must learn how to learn for a lifetime of practice so that current evidence is considered and patient outcomes are optimized.

REFERENCES

1. Bader JD, Shugars DA. Variation in dentists' clinical decisions. *J Public Health Dent.* 1995;55:181–188.
2. Committee on Quality of Health Care in America, IOM. *Crossing the Quality Chasm: A New Health System for the 21st Century.* Washington, DC: The National Academy of Sciences; 2000.
3. Verdonschot E, Angmar-Mansson B, ten Bosch J, et al. Developments in caries diagnosis and their relationship to treatment decisions and quality of care. ORCA Saturday Afternoon Symposium 1997. *Caries Res.* 1999;33:32–40.
4. Bogacki R, Hunt R, Aguila MD, et al. Survival analysis of posterior restorations using an insurance claims database. *Oper Dent.* 2002;27:488–492.
5. Evidence-based Medicine Working Group. Evidence-based medicine: a new approach to teaching the practice of medicine. *JAMA.* 1992;268:2420–2425.
6. Sackett D, Straus S, Richardson W. *Evidence-Based Medicine: How to Practice & Teach EBM.* 2nd ed. London, England: Churchill Livingstone; 2000.
7. Evidence-based Medicine Working Group. *Users' Guides to the Medical Literature, A Manual for EB Clinical Practice.* Chicago: AMA; 2002.
8. Sackett D, Richardson W, Rosenberg W, et al. *Evidence-based Medicine: How to Practice and Teach EBM.* New York: Churchill Livingston; 1997.
9. *Testimony On Health Care Quality.* John Eisenberg, MD, Administrator, AHCPR, before the House Subcommittee on Health and the Environment, October 28, 1997. Agency for Health Care Policy and Research, Rockville, MD. http://www.ahrq.gov/news/test1028.htm
10. Institute of Medicine. *Dental Education at the Crossroads, Challenges and Change.* Washington, DC: National Academy Press; 1995.
11. Bader J, Shugars D. Variation, treatment outcomes, and practice guidelines in dental practice. *J Dent Educ.* 1995;59:61–95.
12. Ecenbarger W. How honest are dentists? *Reader's Dig.* 1997;50–56.
13. Yingling N, Byrne B, Hartwell G. Antibiotic use by members of the American Association of Endodontists in the year 2000: report of a national survey. *J Endod.* 2002;28:396–404.
14. Epstein J, Chong S, Le N. A survey of antibiotic use in dentistry. *J Am Dent Assoc.* 2000;131:1600–1609.
15. Anderson G, Allison D. Intrapartum electronic fetal heart rate monitoring: a review of current status for the Task Force on the Periodic Health Examination. In: *Preventing Disease. Beyond the Rhetoric.* New York: Springer-Verlag, 1990; 19–26.
16. Crowley P, Chalmers I, Keirse M. The effects of corticosteroid administration before preterm delivery: an overview of the evidence from controlled trials. *Br J Obstet Gynecol.* Blackwell Publishing, 1990;97:11–25.
17. Frazier P, Horowitz A. *Prevention: A Public Health Perspective. Oral Health Promotion and Disease Prevention.* Copenhagen, Denmark: Munksgaard; 1995.
18. Grimes DA. Graduate education. *Evid Based Med.* 1995;86:451–457.
19. Sullivan F, MacNaughton R. Evidence in consultations: interpreted and individualised. *Lancet.* 1996;348:941–943.
20. Hall E. Physical therapists in private practice: information sources and information needs. *Bull Med Libr Assoc.* 1995;83:196–201.
21. Gravois S, Bowen D, Fisher W, et al. Dental hygienists' information seeking and computer application behavior. *J Dent Educ.* 1995;59:1027–1033.
22. Curtis K, Weller A. Information-seeking behavior: a survey of health sciences faculty use of indexes and databases. *Bull Med Libr Assoc.* 1993;81:383–392.
23. Ramsey P, Carline J, Inui T. Changes over time in the knowledge base of practicing internists. *JAMA.* 1991;266:1103–1107.
24. Richards D. Which journals should you read to keep up to date? *Evid Based Dent.* 1998;1:22–25.
25. Davidoff F, Case K, Fried P, et al. Evidence-based medicine: why all the fuss? *Ann Intern Med.* 1995;122:727.
26. Forrest J, Horowitz A, Shmuely Y. Caries preventive knowledge and practices among dental hygienists. *J Dent Hyg.* 2000;74:183–195.
27. Niederman R, Chen L, Murzyn L, et al. Benchmarking the dental randomized controlled literature on MEDLINE. *Evid Based Med.* 2002;3:5–9.
28. Forrest JL, Miller S. A bibliometric study of research related to clinical dental hygiene practice. Unpublished research report, 2006.
29. Marsa L. Studies in confusion; knowing what constitutes good research can help consumers evaluate conflicting reports and claims that sound too good to be true. *Los Angeles Times.* April 30, 2001:S.1–5.
30. BBC News. Thumbs down for electric toothbrush. BBC News, World Edition, Health Web site. http://news.bbc.co.uk/2/hi/health/2679175.stm. Accessed March 18, 2007.
31. Stein R. Electric toothbrush tops study—other devices no better than manual kind, researchers say. *Washington Post.* January 12, 2003:A06.
32. Berthold M. Are power toothbrushes better? *ADA News.* January 20, 2003.
33. Rainie L, Packel D. *More Online, Doing More: 16 Million Newcomers Gain Internet Access in the Last Half of 2000 as Women, Minorities, and Families with Modest Incomes Continue to Surge Online.* Washington DC: The Pew Internet & American Life Project. Pew Internet Project: Internet tracking report; 2001.
34. Fincham A, Shuler C. The changing face of dental education: the impact of PBL. *J Dent Educ.* 2001;65:406–421.
35. Pew Health Professions Commission. *Critical Challenges: Revitalizing the Health Professions for the Twenty-First Century.* San Francisco, CA: UCSF Center for the Health Professions; 1995.
36. Forrest JL. Treatment plan for integrating evidence-based decision making into dental education. *J Evid Base Dent Pract.* 2006;6:72–78.
37. Deshpande N, Publicover M, Basford P, et al. Incorporating the views of obstetric clinicians in implementing evidence-supported labour and delivery suite ward rounds: a case study. *Health Info Libr J.* 2003;20:86–94.
38. Werb S, Matear D. Implementing evidence-based practice in undergraduate teaching clinics: a systematic review and recommendations. *J Dent Educ.* 2004;68:995–1003.
39. Ghali W, Staitz R, Eskew A, et al. Successful teaching in evidence-based medicine. *Med Educ.* 2000;34:18–22.

40. Coomarasamy A, Khan K. What is the evidence that postgraduate teaching in evidence based medicine changes anything? A systematic review. *BMJ*. 2004;329:1017–1022.

41. Sackett D, Straus S. Finding and applying evidence during clinical rounds: the "evidence cart." *JAMA*. 1998;280:1336–1368.

42. American Dental Association. ADA Policy on Evidence-based Dentistry. Professional Issues and Research, ADA Guidelines, Positions and Statements. American Dental Association Web site. 2002. www.ada.org/prof/prac/issues/statements/evidencebased.html. Accessed September 7, 2006.

43. American Dental Association Commission on Dental Accreditation. *Accreditation Standards for Dental Education Programs*. Chicago: ADA, 2002.

44. ADEA Center for Educational Policy and Research. Competencies for the New Dentist (as approved by the 1997 House of Delegates). *J Dent Educ*. 2003;67:1–3.

45. ADEA Center for Educational Policy and Research. Recommendations from the ADEA Forum on the predoctoral dental curriculum. Updated March 11, 2005. ADEA Web site. http://www.adea.org/cepr/Documents/Forum%20on%20the%20Predoc%20Dental%20Curric-Rec.pdf. Accessed January 8, 2008.

46. American Dental Education Association. Compendium of curriculum guidelines for allied dental education programs. ADEA Web site. www.adea.org/CEPRWeb/Compendium/Dental_Hygiene_Curriculum_Guidelines.pdf. Accessed September 7, 2006.

47. Hujoel PP, Cunha-Cruz J, Banting DW, et al. Dental flossing and interproximal caries: a systematic review. *J Dent Res*. 2006;85:298–305.

48. Patton LL, Siegel MA, Benoliel R, et al. Management of burning mouth syndrome: systematic review and management recommendations. *Oral Surg Oral Med Oral Pathol Oral Radiol Endod*. 2007;103(Suppl):S39.e1–S39.e13.

SUGGESTED ACTIVITIES

At this time, complete the Quiz below. After completing the Quiz, answer the critical thinking questions. Then, complete Exercise 1-1, which will introduce you to Gail, a patient whose case scenario will be used as an example throughout this book.

QUIZ

1. Define Evidence-Based Practice.

   _____

   _____

2. State the purpose of EBDM.

   _____

   _____

3. All of the following reasons have contributed to the need of EBDM except:
   a. variations in practice patterns.
   b. delays in adopting useful procedures.
   c. increasing access to relevant clinical findings.
   d. practicing as you were taught in school.
   e. providing effective patient care.

4. Explain why the statement, "EBDM relies only on research," is incorrect.

   _____

   _____

   _____

5. Which of the following elements demonstrate that EBDM has come of age?
   a. ADA accreditation standards for dental education
   b. ADEA competencies for dental and dental hygiene education
   c. Evidence-based journals
   d. ADA has defined EBD
   e. All of the above

6. Place the letter of the following steps in the EBDM process in the correct order (steps 1 through 5).

Order 1st → 5th	Steps
2	a. Finding the best evidence
4	b. Applying the results to patient care
1	c. Asking a good clinical question
5	d. Evaluating the results
3	e. Critically appraising the evidence

7. List two benefits of EBDM.

   a. _____

   b. _____

CRITICAL THINKING QUESTIONS

1. Describe a situation when the EBDM process would have been helpful in finding answers for a question.

_____
_____
_____
_____
_____
_____

2. Discuss how EBDM influences dental and dental hygiene practice today.

_____
_____
_____
_____
_____
_____

3. Compare and contrast traditional curricula to evidence-based curricula.

_____
_____
_____
_____
_____
_____
_____

NOTES

_____
_____
_____
_____
_____
_____
_____
_____
_____
_____

EXERCISE 1-1: INTRODUCTION TO GAIL

Gail is a friendly and creative patient who reports mild depression, fibromyalgia, and chronic pain. She is taking numerous medications and at her appointment today is complaining about her mouth. "It is constantly dry. I can't drink enough water. Chewing gum and sucking on candy or lozenges helps a little, but it doesn't provide relief. I have tried rinsing with mouthwash, too, and nothing I do seems to help. It really bothers me. What can I do?"

Upon examination, you find that there is no infection or oral lesions and verify that she does not have Sjögren syndrome. You review Gail's medical history and discuss her most recent medication regimen. Her current medication is the most accurate evidence-based treatment and is appropriate for her conditions. You conclude that the dry mouth is caused from the side effects of her antidepressants and pain medications. Knowing that she cannot discontinue the use of her current medications and that she has already tried gum and lozenges, you set out to find a solution for Gail.

Task

Describe the rationale for the EBDM process for Gail. What is her main concern?

_____

_____

_____

_____

_____

_____

_____

_____

_____

_____

_____

_____

_____

_____

_____

_____

_____

_____

_____

_____

_____

_____

_____

_____

_____

CHAPTER 2

PICO: Asking Good Questions

SKILL 1

Converting Information Needs/Problems into Clinical Questions So That They Can Be Answered.

PURPOSE

The purpose of this section is to discuss PICO-population (P), intervention (I), comparison (C), and outcome(s), a systematic process for converting information needs and problems into clinical questions so that they can be answered. This is a fundamental step in evidence-based decision making (EBDM) because it forces the questioner to focus on the most important single issue and outcome and facilitates the selection of key terms to be used in the computerized search. It also forces a clear identification of the problem, results, and outcomes related to the specific care provided to that patient. Case scenarios outline the sequential steps in this process and demonstrate the application of the skills involved.

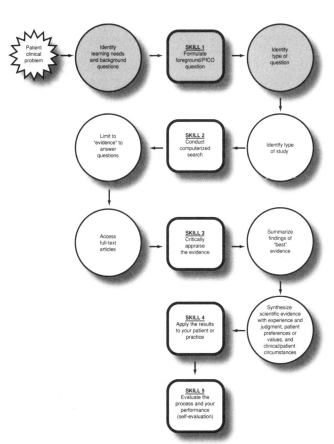

OBJECTIVES

After completing this chapter, the reader will be able to:

1. Identify characteristics of background and foreground questions.
2. Given examples of questions, accurately identify the question as either being a background or foreground question.
3. Given case scenarios, accurately identify the four PICO components of a foreground question and write it out in an appropriate question format.
4. Given a clinical question, rewrite the question as a foreground/PICO question that includes all four PICO components in the appropriate PICO question format.
5. Identify key characteristics of four types of foreground/PICO questions (i.e., therapy, harm, prognosis, diagnosis).
6. Given examples of the four types of foreground/PICO questions, accurately identify the question as therapy, harm, prognosis, or diagnosis.

SUGGESTED ACTIVITIES

Quiz
Critical Thinking Questions
Exercise 2 1
Exercise 2-2

A QUESTION FOR GAIL

EBDM is best learned by actively completing each step in the process. To effectively facilitate this, a case scenario of a patient named Gail will be used as an example in each section and can be used as a template when completing each of the case exercises. Therefore, it is important to introduce Gail.

Gail is a friendly and creative patient who reports mild depression, fibromyalgia, and chronic pain. She is taking numerous medications and at her appointment today is complaining about her mouth. "It is constantly dry. I can't drink enough water. Chewing gum and sucking on candy or lozenges helps a little, but it doesn't provide relief. I have tried rinsing with mouthwash too and nothing I do seems to help. It really bothers me. What can I do?"

During examination, you find that there is no infection or oral lesions and verify that she doesn't have Sjögren syndrome. You review Gail's medical history and discuss her most recent medication regimen. Her current medication is the most accurate evidence-based treatment appropriate for her conditions. You conclude that the dry mouth is caused from the side effects of her antidepressants and pain medications. Knowing she cannot discontinue the use of her current medications and that she has already tried gum and lozenges, you set out to find a solution for Gail.

BACKGROUND AND FOREGROUND QUESTIONS

Background questions are general knowledge inquiries that ask who, what, where, when, how, or why. They are used to help narrow a broad scope and search about a topic to find the details needed for a foreground (PICO) question. A background question may be necessary to identify specific interventions for a disease or problem or to learn more about one particular disorder, intervention, or drug therapy. These questions are helpful in identifying articles that provide more specific details that can be used in developing foreground questions. Finding a good article that reviews the management of a problem often provides the necessary details. In this case, a great article that addresses some of the background questions is "An update of the etiology and management of xerostomia" by Porter et al.[4] Example questions that relate to the Gail case include the following.

- What causes xerostomia?
- What minimizes drug-induced dry mouth?
- What are saliva substitutes?
- What are saliva stimulants?
- What are specific saliva substitutes that are effective for decreasing dry mouth?
- What are specific saliva stimulants that are effective for decreasing dry mouth?
- How are xerostomia patients managed?
- What are the suggested therapies for drug-induced xerostomia?

In completing an Internet PubMed search (which will be outlined in Chapter 5) using the background questions, several specific therapies can be identified that narrow down the broad interventions of saliva stimulants and saliva substitutes. Several studies were identified that might answer Gail's question. These studies address pilocarpine, bethanechol, Cevimeline, anethole trithione—the mucin-containing oral spray Saliva Orthana, and one study that compares eight xerostomia therapies—five saliva stimulants (Salivin, V6, Mucidan, Ascoxal-T, and nicotinamide) and three saliva substitutes (Saliment, Salisynt, and an ex tempore solution). For this case, pilocarpine (a saliva stimulant) and bethanechol (also a saliva stimulant) were selected as therapies for the foreground question. However, keep in mind that any combination of the saliva substitutes or saliva stimulants could be used for Gail.

A foreground question often arises from a problem or client question. It is a specific question that is structured to find a precise answer and phrased to facilitate a computerized search. A "well-built" or foreground question should include four parts that identify the patient problem or PICO.[1] This question is often generated directly by the patient or the care being considered for that patient. However, it can also emerge from an observed problem, a topic of interest, or to explore a new material or procedure, to clarify differences, or compare cost-effectiveness.[2] Foreground or PICO questions are the first step in finding valid evidence to answer a clinical question (Table 2–1).

A preliminary foreground question in Gail's case may be "For a patient with drug-induced dry mouth, will saliva substitutes as compared to saliva stimulants increase salivary flow and decrease dry mouth?" However, saliva substitutes and saliva stimulants is a very broad topic. By using those topics as background questions it is easy to narrow down the terms to specific therapies.

PICO PROCESS

The PICO process was developed as a means for converting information needs and problems into clinical questions so that they can be answered, the first step in the EBDM approach. *Asking the right question is perhaps the hardest skill to learn, and yet it is fundamental to the EBDM process.* The formality of using PICO to frame the question serves three key purposes.

1. It forces the questioner to focus on what the patient/client believes to be the most important single issue and outcome.
2. It facilitates the next step in the process, the computerized search, by selecting language or key terms that will be used in the search.[1]
3. It forces a clear identification of the problem, results, and outcomes related to the specific care provided to that patient. This, in turn, helps to determine the type of evidence and information required to solve the problem and to measure the effectiveness of the intervention.

TABLE 2-1

Differences Between Background and Foreground Questions

Background Question	Foreground Question
General knowledge, broad	Specific
Ask who, what, where, when, how, or why	Identify P, I, C, O
Help narrow a broad scope	Structured to find a precise answer and phrased to facilitate a computerized search
Identify articles that provide more specific details to a broad question	Identify valid evidence to answer a specific question

PICO: population (P), intervention (I), comparison (C), and outcome(s).

One of the greatest difficulties in developing each aspect of the PICO question is providing an adequate amount of information without being too detailed. It is important to stay focused on the main components that directly affect the situation. Each component of a PICO question should be specific, but not merely a laundry list of everything regarding that problem or patient. Each component of the PICO question should be stated as a concise short phrase. This is illustrated in Table 2–2.

PATIENT PROBLEM

The first step in developing a well-built question is to identify the patient problem or population. This is done by describing either the patient's chief complaint or by generalizing the patient's condition to a larger popula-

tion. It is helpful to consider the following when identifying the *P* in PICO.

- How would you describe a group/population with a problem similar to your patient's?
- How you would describe the patient/population to a colleague?
- What are the most important characteristics of this patient/population?
  - Primary problem
  - Patient's main concern or chief complaint
  - Disease (including severity) or health status
  - Age, race, gender, previous ailments, current medications
  - Should these characteristics be considered as I search for evidence?[1]

For some foreground questions, it may be most appropriate to identify a general population instead of

TABLE 2-2

PICO Components for Gail and Three Additional Patient Examples

	Patient/Problem/Population	Intervention	Comparison	Outcome
Gail	Drug-induced xerostomia or xerostomia or drug-induced dry mouth or dry mouth	Pilocarpine	Bethanechol	Increase salivary flow and decrease her perception of dry mouth
Malory	Burning mouth syndrome	Antidepressants	Alpha-lipoic acid	Prevent or minimize the burning sensation on the lips, tongue, or in the mouth
Gavin	Tetracycline staining	Chairside bleaching	At-home professional bleaching	Decrease stain and increase tooth whiteness
Logan	Moderate plaque accumulation	Powered toothbrush	Manual toothbrush	Remove plaque

PICO: population (P), intervention (I), comparison (C), and outcome(s).

focusing on a patient or chief complaint. Examples of populations that may be investigated for a specific case are dental educators, dentists, and menopausal or pregnant women. However, for Gail, the P is a *patient problem* that could be described as "drug-induced xerostomia," "xerostomia," or "drug-induced dry-mouth" or "dry mouth."

The *P* phrase could be more detailed if the added information influences the results of the search. These additional items may include such characteristics as age, gender, health history, or medications. For example, it may be necessary to define the patient as an *adult* in the case of periodontitis or a middle-aged female if the results are regarding postmenopausal women. However, it is usually easier to keep each component as basic as possible so as not to exclude relevant citations when searching the literature. The specific characteristics of the *P* phrase are helpful when appraising the literature and then applying the findings to patients to verify that the studies are applicable and appropriate.

INTERVENTION

Identifying the intervention is the second step in the PICO process. It is important to identify what you plan to *do* for that patient. This may include the use of a specific diagnostic test, treatment, adjunctive therapy, medication, or the recommendation to the patient to use a product or procedure. The intervention is the *one* main consideration for that patient or client.[1] In Gail's case, the main intervention to consider could be pilocarpine based on the findings from the background questions.

COMPARISON

The third phase of the well-built question is the comparison, which is the main intervention alternative being considered.[1] It should be specific and limited to *one* alternative choice to facilitate an effective computerized search. The comparison is the only optional component in the PICO question. Often, one may only look at the intervention without exploring alternatives, and in some cases, there may not be an alternative. For Gail, a comparison could be bethanechol. Often the gold standard is the comparison, especially if a new therapy is being considered.

OUTCOME

The final aspect of the PICO question is the outcome. This specifies the result(s) of what you plan to accomplish, improve, or affect. Outcomes should be *measurable* and may consist of relieving or eliminating specific symptoms, improving or maintaining function, or enhancing esthetics. Specific outcomes also will yield better search results. When defining the outcome, *more effective* is not acceptable unless it describes *how* the intervention is more effective (e.g., more effective in decreasing caries incidence or more effective in preventing tooth fractures). The outcome that we are hoping to achieve for Gail is to increase salivary flow and decrease her perception of dry mouth.

WRITING THE PICO QUESTION

After understanding the elements of PICO, and identifying the patient's concerns, one is now ready to write out the PICO question. Writing out the question is helpful when discussing the components with the patient as well as others involved in providing care. This process also is used when teaching EBDM or consulting with colleagues because it combines all of the essential elements into one concise question that can be investigated and answered. In addition, it is helpful when identifying the four types of questions that will be discussed later in this chapter (Table 2–3).

P—Patient Problem or Population

The first part of the PICO question begins with the following phrase: *In a patient with . . .* Inserting the patient's chief complaint or condition completes this phrase. The Gail PICO question could begin: *In a patient with xerostomia.* Acceptable alternatives for the *P* in Gail's question could be: *In a patient with drug-induced xerostomia: In a patient with dry-mouth: In a patient with drug-induced dry-mouth.* Using the additional examples, these phrases are as follows: *In a patient with burning mouth syndrome: In a patient with Tetracycline staining: In a patient with plaque.*

I—Intervention

The intervention phrase begins with "will . . ." inserting the main intervention being considered for the patient. For Gail, this phrase could be *"will pilocarpine."* For the additional examples the intervention is written: will anti-depressants, will chairside bleaching, will a powered toothbrush.

C—Comparison

The comparison phrase is stated *as compared to* the main alternative being considered for the patient, provided there is one. The Gail question now reads: In a patient with xerostomia, will pilocarpine as compared with bethanechol. The example comparisons are: as compared to alpha-lipoic acid, as compared with at-home bleaching, and as compared with a manual toothbrush.

TABLE 2-3

Writing a PICO Question for Gail and Three Additional Patient Examples

	Write	Patient/Problem/Population	Write	Intervention	Write	Comparison	Outcome
Gail	In a patient with	Drug-induced xerostomia or xerostomia or drug-induced dry mouth or dry mouth	will	Pilocarpine	As compared with	Bethanechol	Increase salivary flow and decrease her perception of dry mouth
Malory	In a patient with	Burning mouth syndrome	will	Antidepressants	As compared with	Alpha-lipoic acid	Prevent or minimize the burning sensation on the lips, tongue, or in the mouth
Gavin	In a patient with	Tetracycline staining	Will	Chairside bleaching	As compared with	At-home professional bleaching	Decrease stain and increase tooth whiteness
Logan	In a patient with	Moderate plaque accumulation	Will	Powered toothbrush	As compared with	Manual toothbrush	Remove plaque

PICO: population (P), intervention (I), comparison (C), and outcome(s).

Name_____   Topic_____

EBDM Worksheet PART A

Skill 1. Converting Information Needs/Problems Into Clinical Questions So That They Can Be Answered

1. **Write your background questions: general knowledge inquiries that ask who, what, where, when, how, or why that you need to learn more about.**

    1. _____
    2. _____
    3. _____
    4. _____
    5. _____
    6. _____
    7. _____
    8. _____
    9. _____
    10. _____

2. **Summarize the findings from your background questions.**

    1. _____
    2. _____
    3. _____
    4. _____
    5. _____

3. **Define your question using PICO by identifying: problem, intervention, comparison group, and outcomes.** *Your question should be used to help establish your search strategy.*

    Patient/problem _____
    Intervention _____
    Comparison _____
    Outcome _____

4. **Write out your PICO question below.**

    _____
    _____

5. **Identify the type of question/problem appropriate for your patient (circle one).**

    Therapy/Prevention   Diagnosis   Etiology, Causation, or Harm   Prognosis

FIGURE 2–1   Evidence-based decision-making worksheet Part A.

Name_____Topic_____

EBDM Worksheet PART A

Skill 1. Converting Information Needs/Problems Into Clinical Questions So That They Can Be Answered

1. **Write your background questions: general knowledge inquiries that ask who, what, where, when, how, or why that you need to learn more about.**

   1. What causes xerostomia?_____

   2. What minimizes drug-induced dry mouth?_____

   3. What are saliva substitutes?_____

   4. What are saliva stimulants?_____

   5. Are saliva substitutes better than saliva stimulants or vice versa?_____

   6. What are specific saliva substitutes that are effective for decreasing dry mouth?_____

   7. What are specific saliva stimulants that are effective for decreasing dry mouth?_____

   8. How are xerostomia patients managed?_____

   9. What are the suggested therapies for drug-induced xerostomia?_____

   10. _____

2. **Summarize the findings from your background questions.**
   1. Most cases of dry mouth are caused by the failure of the salivary glands to function normally. However, in some people dry mouth occurs even though their salivary glands are normal. Although dry mouth is not a disease itself, it can be a symptom of certain diseases. Dry mouth is also a common side effect of some prescription and over-the-counter medications and medical treatments. Over 500 commonly used drugs can cause the sensation of dry mouth. The main culprits are antihypertensives (for high blood pressure) and antidepressants.
   2. Although there is no single way to treat dry mouth, products such as toothpaste, mouthwash, oral gel and gum are available. There are also a number of steps you can follow to keep teeth in good health and relieve the sense of dryness including stimulating saliva and saliva substitutes.
   3. Saliva Stimulants: Acupuncture, Pilocarpine (Salagen), Sorbitol, Xylitol, Mucin, Bethanechol
   4. Saliva Substitutes: Saliva Orthana, Saliva Substitute, Salivart, Xero-Lube
   5. Suggested therapies for drug-induced xerostomia are pilocarpine and bethanechol

3. **Define your question using PICO by identifying: problem, intervention, comparison group, and outcomes.** *Your question should be used to help establish your search strategy.*

   Patient/Problem   Xerostomia_____
   Intervention   Pilocarpine_____
   Comparison   Bethanechol_____
   Outcome   Increase salivary flow and decrease dry mouth_____

4. **Write out your PICO question below.**
   For a patient with drug-induced xerostomia, will pilocarpine as compared to bethanechol increase salivary flow and decrease dry mouth?_____

5. **Identify the type of question/problem appropriate for your patient (circle one).**

   (Therapy/Prevention)   Diagnosis   Etiology, Causation, or Harm   Prognosis

FIGURE 2–2 Part A of evidence-based decision-making worksheet completed for Gail.

O—Outcome(s)

The outcome(s) are then phrased as *the result you would like to happen.* Based on these four parts, the final PICO question for Gail is stated as: *In a patient with xerostomia, will pilocarpine as compared with bethanechol increase salivary flow and decrease dry mouth?* The example questions can be stated as:

- In a patient with burning mouth syndrome, will an antidepressant as compared to alpha-lipoic acid prevent or minimize the burning sensation on the lips, tongue, or in the mouth?
- In a patient with tetracycline staining, will chairside bleaching as compared with at-home bleaching decrease stain and increase tooth whiteness?
- In a patient with moderate plaque accumulation, will a powered toothbrush as compared with a manual toothbrush consistently remove more plaque?

Following the EBDM worksheet Part A (Fig. 2–1), the next step would be to list any additional terms or phrases related to the already identified PICO. Some of the examples of these were already stated for Gail: dry mouth is synonymous with xerostomia. Also, pilocarpine is the generic name for Salagen. By generating these words, alternative key terms are identified that facilitate finding evidence to answer the question. For example, another way of referring to periodontitis would be "periodontal disease" or "chronic destructive periodontitis." By specifying these before conducting a search, time will be used more efficiently. A completed EBDM worksheet Part A for Gail is shown in Figure 2–2.

INTRODUCTION TO FOUR TYPES OF PICO QUESTIONS

Clinical evidence is primarily derived from questions that address therapy/prevention, diagnosis, harm (also known as etiology or causation), and prognosis. The next step is to identify the type of question that is being asked. This facilitates understanding the type of research studies that will best answer the question. The relationship between the type of question and the type of study will be discussed further in Chapter 3.

Therapy/prevention questions look for answers that determine the effect of treatments that avoid adverse events, improve function and are worth the effort and cost.

Example: In a 55-year-old woman with severe rheumatoid arthritis, will anti–tumor necrosis factor-alpha therapy as compared with celecoxib decrease pain and reduce inflammation?

(In these examples, it is important to state the patient's gender and age because they are both risk factors for the disease.)

Diagnosis questions look for evidence to determine the degree to which a test is reliable and useful. The selection and interpretation of diagnostic methods or tests that establish the power of an intervention to differentiate between those with and without a target condition or disease is the aim of diagnosis questions.

Example: In a 55-year-old woman with pain, swelling, and stiffness in the hands and wrists, will a red blood cell test that measures the erythrocyte sedimentation rate as compared with the C-reactive protein test most accurately identify rheumatoid arthritis?

Harm, etiology, causation questions are used to identify causes of a disease or condition including iatrogenic forms and to determine relationships between risk factors, potentially harmful agents, and possible causes of a disease or condition.

Example: In women with rheumatoid arthritis, does cardiovascular disease increase the likelihood of death?

Prognosis questions look to studies that estimate the clinical course or progression of a disease or condition over time and anticipate likely complications (and prevent them).

Example: In a 55-year-old woman will severe rheumatoid arthritis cause loss of fine motor skills-eliminating her ability to crochet?

CONCLUSION

PICO is a systematic process for converting information needs/problems into clinical questions that define the patient problem, intervention, comparison, and outcome. In addition to understanding how to ask a clinical question, identifying the type of question as therapy, diagnosis, harm, or prognosis helps to identify what is being asked. These steps in asking PICO questions establish a solid groundwork for finding the appropriate scientific evidence to answer the questions.

REFERENCES

1. Sackett D, Richardson W, Rosenberg W, et al. *Evidence-Based Medicine: How to Practice and Teach EBM.* New York: Churchill Livingston; 1997.
2. Richards D. Asking the right question right. *Evid Based Dent.* 2000;2:20–21.
3. Forrest JL, Miller SA. Enhancing your practice through evidence-based decision-making. *J Evid Base Dent Pract.* 2001;1:51–57.
4. Porter SR, Scully C, Hegarty AM. An update of the etiology and management of xerostomia. *Oral Surg Oral Med Oral Pathol Oral Radiol Endod.* 2004;97:28–46.

SUGGESTED ACTIVITIES

At this time, complete the quiz below. After completing the quiz, answer the critical thinking questions. Then, work through Exercises 2-1 and 2-2 to strengthen the first skill of the EBDM process: Converting information needs/problems into clinical questions so that they can be answered.

QUIZ

1. Foreground questions are general knowledge inquiries that ask who, what, where, when, how, or why.
   a. True
   b. False

2. PICO questions are only generated directly from the patient or care being considered for a patient.
   a. True
   b. False

3. A PICO question should contain all of the information regarding that problem or patient.
   a. True
   b. False

4. The *P* phrase could be more detailed if added information such as age, sex, or race influences the results you expect to find.
   a. True
   b. False

5. The only optional component of the PICO question is:
   a. P
   b. I
   c. C
   d. O

6. Match the terms with the most appropriate PICO component

   _____P   A. What you plan to do
   _____I   B. Main concern or chief complaint
   _____C   C. Measurable result
   _____O   D. Alternative

7. Select the most appropriate PICO question.
   a. Is antiseptic mouthwash of essential oils as effective as flossing?
   b. For a patient, is an antiseptic mouthwash of essential oils as compared with flossing as effective?
   c. For mild gingivitis is an antiseptic mouthwash of essential oils as effective as flossing?
   d. For a patient with mild gingivitis, is rinsing with an antiseptic mouthwash of essential oils as compared with flossing as effective in reducing plaque and eliminating gingivitis?

8. Select the question that contains the *O* (of PICO):
   a. For a person with mild gingivitis, is an antiseptic mouthwash of essential oils as effective as flossing?
   b. Is mouthwash as effective as flossing?
   c. For a patient with mild gingivitis, is rinsing with an antiseptic mouthwash of essential oils as compared with flossing as effective in reducing plaque and eliminating gingivitis?
   d. For a patient, is an antiseptic mouthwash of essential oils as compared with flossing as effective?

9. Select the PICO component that is missing or incomplete from this sentence: For a patient with periodontal disease, will antimicrobial therapy (minocycline hydrochloride) in conjunction with scaling and root planing as compared with scaling and root planning alone more effective?
   a. P
   b. I
   c. C
   d. O

10. Match each statement with the appropriate type of question.

    _____ Effect of treatments   A. Harm
    _____ Reliability of a test   B. Diagnosis
    _____ Causes of a disease or condition   C. Therapy
    _____ Clinical course of a disease or condition   D. Prognosis

CRITICAL THINKING QUESTIONS

1. Briefly write about a situation, topic, or patient problem for which you do not have answers or complete information for. Then, write what you consider to be the Problem, Intervention, Comparison, Outcome. Write out the PICO question to accompany the scenario.

    _____

    _____

    _____

    _____

    _____

    _____

2. Write a background question about a clinical topic that you would like to know more about.

    _____

    _____

    _____

    _____

    _____

    _____

3. Write a foreground (PICO) question about the same topic from question 2.

    _____

    _____

    _____

    _____

    _____

    _____

4. Discuss how foreground questions are useful in finding answers to clinical questions.

    _____

    _____

    _____

    _____

    _____

    _____

EXERCISE 2-1

Define each PICO component, identifying what is wrong with the question based on the PICO descriptions discussed in this chapter. Then write out a correct question using your clinical experience to fill in the appropriate missing components. There may be several different questions based on how individuals correct the missing pieces.

Exercise 2-1 -PICO and type of Question

Step 1: Determine how complete each question is by identifying each component (P, I, C and O) for the question as is.
Step 2: Correct the components that are wrong or missing by writing the correct P, I, C, and O based on the given case information.
Step 3: Provide the rationale for why it needs to be improved. i.e., wrong-explain why, too broad, too narrow, missing, etc.
Step 4: Revise each PICO question as appropriate by using the CORRECTED PICO components.
Step 3: Identify the type of question for each PICO question. An example is provided.

PICO QUESTION and COMPONENTS

Example: QUESTION: For a 32 year-old mother, is bubble gum fluoride just as effective?

Victoria is a 32 year-old mother of three. She is frustrated because her three children do not brush their teeth. She has found however, that they will use the bubble gum fluoride mouth rinse regularly. She wonders if that is just as effective as brushing teeth. She asks you if she can stop hounding her kids to brush as long as they are using the mouth rinse.

PICO FOR QUESTION AS IS	CORRECTED PICO USING CASE	RATIONALE FOR CHANGE
P = 32 year-old mother of three	P= children	**wrong:** she is asking about her kids not herself
I = bubble gum fluoride	I = fluoride mouth rinse	**wrong:** it is the fluoridated mouthrinse NOT flavored fluoride
C =	C = toothbrushing	**missing:** more specifically toothbrusing
O = just as effective	O = effective in reducing plaque and preventing caries	**too broad:** just as effective is not specific enough- need to describe how it is effective

CORRECTED QUESTION: For children is a fluoride mouthrinse as compared to toothbrushing as effective in reducing plaque and preventing caries?

Type of Question: √ Therapy/Prevention   ☐ Diagnosis   ☐ Etiology, Causation, Harm   ☐ Prognosis

1. **QUESTION:** For a female golfer who loves pizza and has oral malodor, will tongue brushing compared to mouth rinsing fix the problem?

Jaime is 27 year old woman who loves to golf. Her favorite food is pizza, however she is bothered by her bad breath after eating it. She is curious what methods are available to help her breath be better. She wants to know if brushing her tongue will help or if she can use an anti-bacterial mouthrinse to fix the problem.

PICO FOR QUESTION AS IS	CORRECTED PICO USING CASE	RATIONALE FOR CHANGE
P = _____	P = _____	_____
I = _____	I = _____	_____
C = _____	C = _____	_____
O = _____	O = _____	_____

CORRECTED QUESTION:

Type of Question: ☐ Therapy/Prevention   ☐ Diagnosis   ☐ Etiology, Causation, Harm   ☐ Prognosis

2. **QUESTION:** For Alex, is an oral brush biopsy (Oral CDx) a good test?

Alex is a 22 year old guy that just moved to town. He has healthy teeth and gums. He recently had a cleaning completed last month at another office. Upon examination you notice a mucosal lesion, which may be cancerous. You have been conducting manual punch biopsies for most suspicious lesions, but recently read about Oral CDx- an oral brush biopsy. You would like to know if this might be a good test for Alex.

PICO FOR QUESTION AS IS
P = _____
I = _____
C = _____
O = _____

CORRECTED PICO USING CASE
P = _____
I = _____
C = _____
O = _____

RATIONALE FOR CHANGE
_____
_____
_____
_____

CORRECTED QUESTION:

Type of Question: ☐ Therapy/Prevention   ☐ Diagnosis   ☐ Etiology, Causation, Harm   ☐ Prognosis

3. **QUESTION:** For a patient with moderate periodontitis, will bacterial endocarditis occur after a periodontal scaling and root planing?

Dustin is a new patient. He reveals that he has a heart murmur with regurgitation. He has moderate periodontitis and hasn't been seen by a dentist in many years. In the past, his specific health condition was pre-medicated with antibiotic prophylaxis. However, new evidence reveals that pre-medication is not necessary. You want to make sure that his having periodontal scaling and root planning won't cause bacterial endocarditis.

PICO FOR QUESTION AS IS
P = _____
I = _____
C = _____
O = _____

CORRECTED PICO USING CASE
P = _____
I = _____
C = _____
O = _____

RATIONALE FOR CHANGE
_____
_____
_____
_____

CORRECTED QUESTION:

Type of Question: ☐ Therapy/Prevention   ☐ Diagnosis   ☐ Etiology, Causation, Harm   ☐ Prognosis

4. **QUESTION:** For a patient who had oral cancer will he get oral cancer again and lose jaw bone?

Alex is a current patient of yours who is in today to have the stitches taken out from where he had a cancerous lesion removed by the oral surgeon. He is glad that you caught the lesion before the cancer progressed to the bone. However, he is concerned that he may get more cancerous lesions that are more progressive and that he may lose jaw bone. He asks you to find out the likelihood of this happening.

PICO FOR QUESTION AS IS
P = _____
I = _____
C = _____
O = _____

CORRECTED PICO USING CASE
P = _____
I = _____
C = _____
O = _____

RATIONALE FOR CHANGE
_____
_____
_____
_____

CORRECTED QUESTION:

Type of Question: ☐ Therapy/Prevention   ☐ Diagnosis   ☐ Etiology, Causation, Harm   ☐ Prognosis

5. **QUESTION:** Can endodontically treated teeth withstand orthodontic treatment?

Aaron is a healthy 19 year-old male who has eight endodontically treated teeth. He would really like to improve his smile and wants to explore the possibility of getting braces. However, he has heard that there is a risk of apical root resorption in the teeth that have had root canals. He thinks he probably shouldn't get braces but would like to know what you think.

PICO FOR QUESTION AS IS	**CORRECTED PICO USING CASE**	**RATIONALE FOR CHANGE**
P = _____	P = _____	_____
I = _____	I = _____	_____
C = _____	C = _____	_____
O = _____	O = _____	_____

CORRECTED QUESTION:

Type of Question: ☐ Therapy/Prevention ☐ Diagnosis ☐ Etiology, Causation, Harm ☐ Prognosis

EXERCISE 2-2

This is a case series that will be used throughout the workbook. Please read the five case examples presented here. Use the EBDM Worksheet Part A to write background questions & then summarize your findings. Then identify the PICO components and write out the PICO question for each case. Finally, identify the type of question being asked after completing this exercise, you should have 5 EBDM Worksheets PART A filled out. Each of these exercises can be completed individually or as a group.

The examples may also be assigned to different pairs that could each complete one together and present the answer to the group. Do not be discouraged if it takes several attempts and some lively discussion to refine the PICO elements before you have a clearly stated question. With practice, it will become second nature and enhance question writing skills.

Morty

Mr. Morty Kramer is a 55-year-old man who has been using unwaxed floss his whole life and flosses frequently. At his last dental appointment, he was treated by a new hygienist, who told him that he needed to change to a waxed floss because it is more effective in removing plaque. Morty is happy with his current oral hygiene regimen and asks if he really needs to change.

Trevor

Trevor is a 27-year-old bartender who has used chewing tobacco for 13 years. He is a frequent user who chews almost 5 hours a day. He has just learned from his oral health care provider that he has developed precancerous lesions in the vestibular area where he holds the tobacco plug. This new information has motivated him to quit. Trevor knows he can't quit by will power alone because he has tried in the past. He wants to know if a non–nicotine aid in tobacco cessation is helpful in this endeavor or if a nicotine patch is better in helping users permanently quit. He would like to know if behavioral therapy/counseling might help.

Dr. Bailer

Dr. Bailer recently graduated from dental school and is building a new dental practice. As he designs his building, he is trying to decide whether to purchase digital radiograph equipment or to use traditional radiography. He is interested in knowing the most accurate method for caries detection.

Jennifer

Your morning patient, Mrs. Jennifer Morris, comes to you distressed because of an article she read on the Internet about the dangers of mercury in her amalgam restorations. She is worried that her seven amalgam fillings are poisoning her. She is very concerned not only for her own health, but for her two young daughters who also have amalgam restorations. Jennifer doesn't want to replace her fillings if it isn't necessary, but needs proof that she and her children are going to be healthy.

To reassure your patient, you give her advice based on your clinical experience and judgment; however, she still seems very upset and troubled. You inform her that you will investigate the latest information and get back to her with your findings. She seems more relaxed with this thought and leaves eager to hear from you soon.

Sam

Sam is a 49-year-old man with moderate periodontitis, who was recently diagnosed with type 2 diabetes mellitus. Sam's glycosylated hemoglobin is 12%, which places him in the category of poorly controlled diabetes. Sam is worried that his diabetes will increase his chance of losing his teeth. He wants to know the effect and impact diabetes now has on his oral health.

Name_____Topic_____

EBDM Worksheet PART A

*Skill 1. Converting Information Needs/Problems Into Clinical Questions So That They
         Can Be Answered*

1. **Write your btackground questions: general knowledge inquiries that ask who, what,
   where, when, how, or why that you need to learn more about.**

   1. _____

   2. _____

   3. _____

   4. _____

   5. _____

   6. _____

   7. _____

   8. _____

   9. _____

   10. _____

2. **Summarize the findings from your background questions.**

   1. _____

   2. _____

   3. _____

   4. _____

   5. _____

3. **Define your question using PICO by identifying: problem, intervention, comparison group,
   and outcomes.** *Your question should be used to help establish your search strategy.*

   Patient/problem ——————————————————————————
   Intervention ————————————————————————————
   Comparison ————————————————————————————
   Outcome ——————————————————————————————

4. **Write out your PICO question below.**

   _____
   _____

5. **Identify the type of question/problem appropriate for your patient (circle one).**

   Therapy/Prevention   Diagnosis   Etiology, Causation, or Harm   Prognosis

CHAPTER 3

Research Design and Sources of Evidence

PURPOSE

The purpose of this section is to discuss sources of scientific evidence and characteristics of research designs that constitute the evidence. Although evidence-based decision making (EBDM) emphasizes using randomized clinical trials and other quantifiable methods, this focus has evolved to include qualitative research and acknowledging that different research designs contribute to a continuum of knowledge.

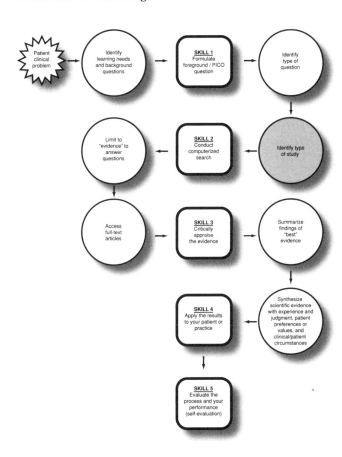

OBJECTIVES

After completing this chapter, readers will be able to:

1. Identify what constitutes evidence.
2. Explain the difference between research and evidence.
3. Identify sources of primary and secondary evidence.
4. Discuss the difference between experimental and non-experimental research.

5. Identify distinguishing characteristics of different research methods: randomized control, cohort, case control, case series, and case report studies.
6. Discuss the difference between quantitative and qualitative research and the role of qualitative research in EBDM.
7. Identify scientific sources of evidence to use in clinical decision making.

SUGGESTED ACTIVITIES

Quiz
Critical Thinking Questions
Exercise 3-1

SOURCES OF EVIDENCE

Scientific evidence is the product of well-designed and well-controlled research investigations that minimize sources of bias. Evidence is considered the synthesis of all valid research studies that answer a specific question. As such, a single research study does not constitute "the evidence," but rather contributes to a body of knowledge that has been derived from multiple studies investigating the same phenomena.[1] Thus, the body of evidence evolves over time as more research is conducted, underscoring the importance of staying current with the scientific literature. Once synthesized, evidence can help inform decisions about whether a method of diagnosis or a treatment is effective relative to other diagnostic methods or treatment and under what circumstances. The challenge in using EBDM arises when there is only *one* research study available on a particular topic. In these cases, individuals should be cautious in relying on the study because later it can be contradicted by another study or have used poor methods or it may only test efficacy (safety and how well an intervention performs under ideal conditions) and not effectiveness (how well an intervention works in everyday practice).

Historically, traditional sources of evidence included printed materials such as textbooks, personal journal collections, conference proceedings, and clinical guidelines, which may or may not have been based on well-conducted research. Colleagues, mentors, those considered experts in the field, and personal experiences also were a predominant source of information for treatment decisions.[2–4] However, many of these sources fall into weaker categories of evidence, or are not even considered evidence because they do not use a scientific process or a structured method for making objective observations. As health professions have adopted EBDM, they have increasingly emphasized use of sources of evidence that reduce bias. It is important to recognize that, in addition to support through scientific investigations or when there are no studies that address the specific question, the EBDM process also includes the clinician's experience and judgment, the patient's values and preferences, and the clinical circumstances. EBDM seeks to blend experience and values with best evidence.

There are two types of evidence-based sources: primary and secondary. **Primary sources** are original research publications that have not been filtered or synthesized, such as individual research articles. Primary research consists of both quantitative and qualitative research. Most of the research and literature related to EBDM refers to **quantitative research,** which focuses on establishing cause-and-effect relationships through testing a specific hypothesis and reporting the results in statistical terms. In comparison, **qualitative research** is exploratory and uses an interpretive, naturalistic approach that focuses on how individuals or groups view and understand their surroundings and construct meaning out of their experiences. Qualitative research investigates the why and how of decision making, and data are typically reported using narrative terms and not displayed mathematically in tables or graphs. For example, some participants in a focus group on oral cancer prevention and early detection reported, "They checked the inside of my cheeks and pulled out my tongue and felt my neck. They didn't tell me what they were doing."[5] Table 3-1 summarizes the characteristics of quantitative and qualitative research approaches. Additional discussion is provided in the chapters that follow.

QUANTITATIVE PRIMARY RESEARCH: EXPERIMENTAL STUDIES

Experimental studies are those in which the researcher controls or manipulates the variables under investigation, such as in testing the effectiveness of a treatment. These studies are the most complex and include randomized controlled trials and controlled clinical trials.

Randomized Controlled Trial

The **randomized controlled trial** (RCT) provides the strongest evidence for demonstrating cause and effect (i.e., the treatment has caused the effect, rather than it happening by chance). An RCT study design involves the following.

- At least one test/experimental treatment or intervention and one control treatment that can be a placebo treatment or no treatment.
- Concurrent enrollment of subjects and follow-up of the experimental test- and control-treated groups.
- Assignment of subjects to either the experimental treatment/intervention group or the control/placebo group through a random process, such as the use of a random-numbers table.
- Follow-up of both groups to determine the outcome.

The most important characteristics of RCTs are the ability to randomly assign subjects to either the experimental or control group and to randomly allocate treatments. Other unique features of RCTs that reduce bias and strengthen validity are that they are prospective in nature and can include blind or double blind strategies. A **double-blind RCT** is one in which neither the patient nor the investigator knows whether the patient is receiving the experimental treatment or the control treatment. Studies involving therapies (pills/liquids/pastes) are easy to double-blind because the subject takes one of two treatments of identical size/dose, shape, and color, and neither the patient nor the investigator knows who is taking the treatment or the placebo. It is more difficult to double-blind studies when testing a new treatment, technique, or procedure in which the investigator or patient can distinguish a difference. In these studies, an examiner who has not been involved in the implementation of the study should be used to evaluate the results to decrease bias.

Nonrandomized Clinical Trials

Nonrandomized clinical trials often rely on historical controls that cannot establish true equivalence so that there is less confidence in the findings. For example, in cancer research, patients receive a new treatment and their responses are compared with controls from previous studies; however, the controls may not provide a good comparison depending on how long ago the study was conducted, or differences in treatment, technology, and patient care that have occurred since that time.[8]

Nonrandomized clinical trials also are used to screen new therapies. The purpose is not to prove the treatment is efficacious, but that there is sufficient activity to be tested in a randomized study. These studies require fewer patients; however, they are subject to investigator and placebo bias because all patients are treated in an unblinded manner.[8] Finally, nonrandomized clinical trials, or **controlled trials**, may be used in diagnostic studies in which the outcomes from a new test under evaluation are compared with outcomes from the reference or **gold standard test** (i.e., the test or measure considered the ultimate or ideal). In controlled trials, there is no

TABLE 3-1

Characteristics of Quantitative and Qualitative Research Approaches[6,7]

	Quantitative		Qualitative
	Experimental	*Nonexperimental*	*Nonexperimental*
Purpose and study design	Begins with hypothesis and tests cause and effect; variables are defined and manipulated. Answers questions related to therapy and harm in terms of how many or how much; probability sampling allows generalizing findings, uses a deductive process Double- or single-blinded RCTs or nonblinded RCTs or controlled trials	Observational studies used to systematically describe and interpret conditions/relationships that already exist. Examines the association between a particular exposure and a risk factor; or between a disease and hypothesized risk factors. A treatment or intervention is not given Cohort, case control and case series, or report studies	Uses a naturalistic approach to answer questions about the meaning, or attitudes, beliefs, or behavior of a group or individual; provides explanation and understanding; uses an inductive process; used to generate hypotheses Phenomenology, ethnography, and grounded theory
Data collection	Systematic data collection using predefined methods of measurement. Often have blinding of examiners to minimize bias when examining experimental and control groups	Gathers data without giving a treatment or intervening to control variables; clinical exam, survey, or questionnaires. Can be collected once or multiple times over time	Fieldwork to observe people and record in the natural setting. Data collected via focus groups, observation, unstructured interviews, diaries, written anecdotes, philosophy, poetry, or art
Role of researcher	Tends to remain separate from the subject matter		Tends to be immersed in the subject matter; personal involvement
Analysis	Analysis occurs after all data are collected. Involves analysis of numerical data that can be combined and manipulated using statistical methods. Results reported using numerical relations and statistical terms		Analysis takes place concurrently with data collection and is ongoing. Involves analysis of thoughts or concepts, pictures, or objects and categorized into themes. Reported in narrative terms

randomization because *both tests are given to all individuals* who are suspected of having the condition of interest, and measurements from each test are compared to determine if the new test is as accurate as the reference or gold standard test.[9]

QUANTITATIVE PRIMARY RESEARCH

Nonexperimental Studies

Nonexperimental studies are those in which the researcher does not give a treatment, intervention, or provide an exposure (i.e., data is gathered without intervening to control variables). Examples of nonexperimental studies include cohort studies, case control studies, case series, and case reports.

Cohort Studies

Cohort studies make observations about the association between a particular exposure or a risk factor (e.g., tobacco use) and the subsequent development of a disease or condition (e.g., lung cancer). In these studies, subjects do not presently have the condition of interest (lung cancer) and are followed over time to see at what frequency they develop the disease/condition as compared with a control group who is not exposed to the risk factor (tobacco use) under investigation (Fig. 3-1).

As in experimental studies, both groups are followed prospectively and there is the ability to establish

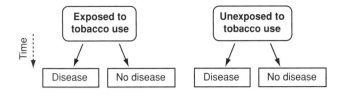

Persons *with and without the* **exposure** of interest (e.g., tobacco) are identified at the initiation of the study. Information is then collected looking forward in time to identify outcomes (i.e., disease [lung cancer] or no disease). At the start of the study, neither group has the disease or condition of interest.

FIGURE 3–1 Prospective cohort study design.

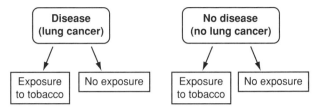

Persons *with and without the* **disease** of interest (e.g., lung cancer) are identified at the initiation of the study. Information is then collected looking backward in time to identify potential exposure or risk factors (e.g., tobacco) that could have contributed to getting the disease.

FIGURE 3–2 Case control—retrospective study design.

a temporal sequence for the relationship between exposure to risk factors and development of a particular disease or condition.[10] The temporal sequence (i.e., the exposure has to precede the development of the disease/condition) is necessary for drawing inferences about causative factors. The important advantage of this design is the ability to control and monitor data collection and to measure variables accurately.

A cohort study is most useful when the disease/condition of interest occurs frequently and subjects can be readily obtained. It also is useful when the risk factors are known or thought to cause harm (tobacco use) and when there are ethical considerations. For example, researchers could not conduct an experimental study to determine if tobacco use causes lung cancer. This would require that subjects (all nonusers of tobacco) be randomly assigned to an experimental or control group and have those in the experimental group start smoking "x" number packs of cigarettes per day. Instead, investigators find people who already smoke "x" number packs of cigarettes per day (and who do not have lung cancer) and match them with as similar a group as possible, with the exception of not smoking, to serve as the control group. Both groups then are followed over time and the incidence of lung cancer in those who smoke is compared with the incidence of lung cancer in those who do not smoke. Obvious disadvantages are the time it could take to develop the disease or condition of interest (lung cancer), the cost of follow-up, and the potential for losing subjects over time.

Case Control Studies

Case control studies make observations about possible associations between the disease of interest (lung cancer) and one or more hypothesized risk factors (tobacco use).[10] Case control studies are retrospective in that subjects *already have a certain disease or condition* and are compared with a representative group of disease-free people (controls) from the same population (Fig. 3-2).

A case control study is most useful in studying the etiology of rare diseases because they are difficult to study on a population basis. Also, a case study allows multiple etiologic factors to be studied concurrently.[10]

The problem with case control studies is that investigators are looking back in time and often have to rely on the subjects' recall or other incomplete sources of information for exposure histories or characteristics that could have put a person at risk for developing the condition or disease of interest. The assumption is that the differences should explain why the cases developed the condition/disease of interest and the controls did not. Although simplified, using the tobacco and lung cancer example, lung cancer patients would be asked questions related to their smoking history. For example, do they currently smoke, or have they every smoked and, if so, when did they started smoking, how much do they smoke, when did it increase and by how much; did they ever stop and then start again and when; and their answers would be compared with those of the control group. As a result, this study design lends itself to recall bias and extraneous variables more so than a cohort or experimental study. Case control studies also are less reliable because a statistical relationship between two conditions does not mean that one condition actually caused the other. For instance, lung cancer rates may be higher for people who earn less than $50,000 per year, but that does not mean that someone can reduce his or her cancer risk just by getting a salary increase to more than $50,000. When possible, researchers should confirm the results with a randomized controlled trial or a prospective cohort study.

Case Series and Case Reports

Case series and case reports are often reported in the dental and dental hygiene literature. These consist either of collections of reports on the treatment of several patients, or a report of a single patient. For example, if a patient has a condition that a clinician has never seen or heard of before and is uncertain what to do, a search for case series or case reports may reveal information that will assist in a diagnosis. However, for any reasonably well-known condition, there should be better evidence. Case series and case reports have no statistical validity, because they report observations and do not use a control group with which to compare outcomes. However, they can be extremely important in identifying new health concerns and often generate a hypothesis that then sparks the initiation of more rigorous prospective studies and clinical trials as they did with toxic shock syndrome[11] and AIDS.[12]

QUALITATIVE PRIMARY RESEARCH

Qualitative research is nonexperimental in that it conducts studies in natural settings in an attempt to understand an event from the point of view of the participants. It seeks to provide depth of understanding and does so through answering questions such as what, how, and why. It explores issues in more depth with those experiencing the issue rather than testing a hypothesis to answer questions such as how many or what proportion.

In many cases, qualitative research generates new theory. Also, it complements quantitative research by attempting to clarify the meaning of how many or by providing a greater understanding of why an intervention works. For example, quantitative research may ask, "How many smokers have tried to quit?" whereas qualitative research explores "What stops smokers from quitting?" The most important consideration in designing a study is to use the right methodology to answer the question.

Good qualitative research requires a very rigorous design. Criteria include: stating a clear aim of the research, which includes both context and process, and documenting transferability (a detailed description of the sample and findings so that similarities and differences can be identified); dependability (clear records of the research process and its products); confirmability (conclusions are fair so that there is confidence in the findings; multiple data sources are used); and credibility (internal validity—do the findings make sense).[6]

Qualitative research has many different research designs and data collection methods based on the questions being explored and the setting being observed. Three common study designs include: ethnography, phenomenology, and grounded theory. Ethnography asks, "What is the culture of a group of people?" and collects data through participant observation, unstructured interviews, and studying documents and photographs. Culture is not limited to ethnic groups, but may involve organizations, programs, and groups of people with common social or health problems. Phenomenology answers

the question, "What is it like to have a certain experience?" and collects data through in-depth interviews, written anecdotes, philosophy, poetry, or art. Examples of experiences include those related to emotions, relationships, or to being part of an organization or group. Grounded theory builds on the inductive nature of qualitative research and focuses on theory construction and verification by studying interactions as they occur naturally. Data collection methods include taped interviews, participant observation, focus groups, and diaries. Tables 3-2 and 3-3 provide further information related to the focus of each study design and the correct data gathering method used to generate the data to answer the research objective.

SECONDARY RESEARCH: SYSTEMATIC REVIEWS AND META-ANALYSIS

Secondary research is filtered or synthesized publications of the primary research literature. These sources include systematic reviews (SRs) and meta-analyses, evidence-based article reviews of already conducted research, and evidence-based clinical practice guidelines.

With more than 2 million articles published annually and 20,000 biomedical journals, SRs provide a way of managing large quantities of information[13] by providing a summary of two or more primary research studies that have investigated the same specific phenomenon or question. This scientific technique defines a specific question to be answered and uses explicit predefined criteria for retrieval of studies, assessment, and synthesis of evidence from individual RCTs and other well-controlled methods. Methods used in SRs parallel those of RCTs in that each step is thoroughly documented and reproducible. For example, there are predefined criteria for the inclusion and exclusion of research studies in an SR just as there are predefined criteria for the inclusion and exclusion of subjects in an individual RCT. Figure 3-3 demonstrates how individual research studies contribute to building a body of

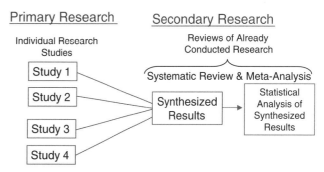

FIGURE 3–3 Differences between primary and secondary sources.

TABLE 3-2

Qualitative Research Paradigms

Criteria → Paradigms (Research Strategy)	Research Questions Guide (but Do not Restrict) the Inquiry	Methods of Data Gathering and Analysis Consistent With Philosophical and Epistemological Traditions from Which They are Derived and are Compatible with the Type of Question being Asked	Methods of Data Gathering and Analysis are Rigorously and Appropriately Applied Describes: How Participants Selected Methods Used to Generate Data Comprehensiveness of Data Collection Procedures for Analyzing Data	Thoughtful and Ethical Plan For Entering the Field of Study; Establishing and Maintaining Relationship and Exiting the Field is Illustrated	Conclusions are Based Upon Research Results. Data Analysis is Systematic and Meaningful.
Phenomenology Describes lived experiences of individuals as interpreted by the researcher. (Philosophy)	What is the meaning of the phenomenon? What is it like to have a certain experience? Can be related to emotions, relationships, part of an organization or group.	In-depth interviews, written anecdotes, philosophy, poetry or art. Experience provided direction of the study.	Presented examples of research questions.	Identified people, the use of art, poetry, etc.	Reflective description of the experience: "What it felt like to. . ." Researcher's bias and influence of their own point of view is stated and discussed within the context of the study
Ethnography Used to study people of other cultures. (Cultural anthropology)	What is the nature of this phenomenon? What is the culture of a group of people? Culture may be an ethnic group, organization, program, group of people with common social or health problems.	Participant observation, unstructured interviews, documents, photographs. Researcher learns from participants the meanings they attach to activities, events, behaviors, rituals, knowledge and lifestyle.		Participants and observers of participants	Description of day-to-day events Researcher's bias and influence of their own point of view is stated and discussed within the context of the study

(Continued)

T A B L E 3 – 2

(Continued)

Criteria → Paradigms (Research Strategy)	Research Questions Guide (but Do not Restrict) the Inquiry	Methods of Data Gathering and Analysis Consistent With Philosophical and Epistemological Traditions from Which They are Derived and are Compatible with the Type of Question being Asked	Methods of Data Gathering and Analysis are Rigorously and Appropriately Applied Describes: How Participants Selected Methods Used to Generate Data Comprehensiveness of Data Collection Procedures for Analyzing Data	Thoughtful and Ethical Plan For Entering the Field of Study, Establishing and Maintaining Relationship and Exiting the Field is Illustrated	Conclusions are Based Upon Research Results. Data Analysis is Systematic and Meaningful.
Grounded Theory Discovers basic patterns in social life to generate theories. Used for conceptualizing. (Sociology)	What are the interactions or processes going on? Does not start with a specific research question. Researcher begins study by looking at underlying social and psychological processes that relate to conditions in a particular setting	Taped interviews, participant observation, focus groups, diaries. Studies interactions as they occur naturally.	Researcher identifies key variable that explains what is occurring and further develops emerging theory. Lit review occurs after researcher identifies emerging theory. Data analysis compares emerging theory with existing research (theories).	Key people who play specific roles	Theory development with respect to social and psychological processes. Theory is developed or reformulated from the existing source. Researcher's bias and influence of their own point of view is stated and discussed within the context of the study.

McMaster; http://www.cche.net/usersguides/qualitative.asp

Mita Giacomini, Deborah J. Cook, for the Evidence Based Medicine Working Group. Based on the Users' Guides to Evidence-based Medicine and reproduced with permission from JAMA. (2000 Jul 26;284(4):478–482) Copyright 2000, American Medical Association.

T A B L E 3 – 3

Qualitative Research Methods

Methods	Rationale	Nature of Research Questions	Sampling No. and Group Composition	Recording Data
Observation Overt or covert	Natural setting; can overcome discrepancy between what is said and what is actually done Want to communicate cultural values of setting Can identify processes of which people are unaware	Answers why; observing working of organizations and how people perform functions Cultures	Purposive; deliberate group or setting; not generalizable; Should select a good representational setting with features and categories relevant to a wide range of settings	Systematic recording of field notes. May ask questions or analyze documents. Looking especially for tentative hypotheses and negative cases.
Interviews 1) Structured-questionnaire 2) Semistructured 3) In depth	Explore people's knowledge, experiences and framework of meanings	To understand practices and discover factors that contribute to situation. How and why phenomena occur	Determined by nature of research; purposive sampling. Statistical representation not sought. Sample size determined by depth and duration of interview and what is feasible Large study may have 50–60 at most	Tape recorder: transcription is time consuming. Field notes at time of interview interferes with process; afterwards may forget or miss some details
Focus Groups Group interviews	Capitalize on communication among participants in order to generate data. Interactions are part of method. Highlight values and norms of culture (e.g., why or why not they use health services).	What people think, how they think and why they think that way. Exploring responses to health education messages; public understanding of health and illness. Health behaviors, experiences with disease and health services; attitudes and needs of staff	Most include few groups; 4–8 people is ideal; 1–2 hours Homogeneous groups capitalize on shared experiences. Existing groups → naturally occurring setting can relate or challenge each other. Theoretical sampling with subjects selected to represent range of total study population or to test hypotheses. Diversity may be needed to explore different perspectives.	Taped and transcribed; series of statements on cards; questionnaire. Group records issues on flip chart

(Continued)

TABLE 3 – 3

(Continued)

Methods	Rationale	Nature of Research Questions	Sampling No. and Group Composition	Recording Data
Case Study 1) Precise questions during data collection and analysis (allows comparisons) 2) Study implemented empirically	Practical and policy questions; health services research (HSR) Understand principles guiding design and conduct of evals; Involves complex mix of changes, different time scales, involvement of different groups (providers, admin); Study implementation of health policies empirically versus analyzing proposed projects analytically Retrospective or prospective	Real life intervention focus Semistructured; ethnography-eventually research questions emerge; research → impact of government policies in health system Forming judgments about appropriateness of an intervention. Investigate how and why it succeeded or failed; whether outputs and outcomes of intervention are justified by their inputs and processes	Sites typical of phenomena being studied Those in which a specific theory can be tested or that will confirm or refute a hypoth; Replication of results across sites → ensure findings not due to site characteristics	Depends on methods chosen. Researchers want to build chains of evidence-conceptual arguments that link phenomena to one another.
Consensus Methods	Method to synthesize info using wider range of information than meta-analysis. Determine extent to which experts or lay people agree about a given issue	When need to make decisions where there is little or conflicting evidence or overload of information. For clarifying issues in organization or defining professional roles	Experts, relevant individuals	Defined structured process for conducting, tabulating and providing results/ratings back to participants
1) Delphi technique	Where published information is inadequate or nonexistent	Unanimity of opinion does not exist owing to lack of scientific evidence or where there is contradictory evidence on an issue	Delphi: conducted by mail	
2) Nominal Group Process	Harness insights of appropriate experts to enable decisions to be made Deriving quantitative estimates through qualitative approaches	Consensus measurement and consensus development	Nominal: conducted in person; 9–12 people	

(Continued)

TABLE 3–3

(Continued)

Methods	Role of Researcher	Analysis or Interpretation	Advantages	Limitations
Observation Overt or covert	Researcher to act as research instrument and documenter necessary that observations are systematically recorded and analyzed: record own feelings and responses to situation witnessed. Needs to be able to establish rapport May be involved in activities while also observing them	Iterative process of developing categories from notes, testing against hypotheses and refining. Basis of tentative hypothesis or evolution of systems classification Not distinct stages but occurs with data collection Validity: truthful and systematic representation of research; communicate culture and rules enough to allow another researcher to learn them and pass as a member of the group	Uncover behavior or routine of which participants may be unaware; overcome discrepancies between what is said and what is done Can build on quantitative research → understanding of why	Researcher behavior immersion Hawthorne effect Gaining access to group Going "native" Large amounts of data to analyze Reliability and validity, generalization Researcher may not observe what they really want to see
Interviews 1) Structured-questionnaires 2) Semistructured 3) Indepth	Discover interviewees own framework of meanings; must avoid imposing own structures and assumptions; remain open to new concepts that may be very different than predicted	Transcription of data after collection; can influence refinement of questions for next interview	Can probe and explore issues in depth to get to the bottom of what you want—better than observation. Can open up new areas of research; investigate questions of immediate relevance	Skills of interviewer; must be sensitive to vocabulary of interviewee; People do not do what they say all the time Problems with recall, bias and selective remembering Hard to categorize and summarize data that researcher has: 1) understood respondent's meaning instead of relying on their own assumptions; 2) the questions are neutral, sensitive, clear

(Continued)

TABLE 3–3

(Continued)

Methods	Role of Researcher	Analysis or Interpretation	Advantages	Limitations
Focus Groups Group interviews	Facilitate interaction among members of the group	Compares discussions of similar themes; distinguish between individual opinion and group consensus. Report deviant cases, minority opinions; impact of group dynamics and interaction between participants	Does not discriminate against people who can not read or write. Encourages participation from people reluctant to be interviewed on their own feelings or believe they have nothing to say. Can empower; safety in numbers.	Can lack confidentiality Dominant views may silence other group members Data analysis is time consuming
Case Study 1) Precise questions during data collection & analysis (allows comparisons) 2) Study implemented empirically	Multiple methods used Semi-structured interviews; focus groups, observations	Multiple methods and sources of evidence to establish construct validity Triangulation: at least 1 other source and usually another method of data collection Explain quantitative findings, e.g., explain why there was an increase or decrease in number of referrals, number of admissions	Complexity of issues—evaluation of health services interventions Answer how and why events take a particular course	Complex Single coherent account of events can vary widely Site selection can be difficult Multiple methods are hard to manage Evaluation to inform policy requires overall judgement of success or failure
Consensus Methods 1) Delphi technique 2) Nominal group process		Agreement: 1) extent to which each respondent agrees with an issue-numerical scale 2) extent to which respondents agree with each other = consensus; average + dispersion	*Delphi:* Confidentiality; One person or coalition is not able to dominate Iterative process allows participants to change minds Controlled feedback Statistical group responses Large number of experts can be contacted cheaply	Justification of these methods Potential for bias in selection of experts. Difficult to define "acceptable" levels. Typical disadvantage of group decision-making. Presentation of findings; testing findings against observed data.

knowledge[14] and the difference between primary and secondary sources.

Systematic reviews differ from traditional literature or narrative reviews in that they are narrower in scope and focus on answering specific questions. Those conducting SRs try to find all the literature addressing a specific question, including unpublished or **"gray" literature**. The gray literature may include reports, working papers, theses/dissertations, government documents, conference proceedings, or meeting abstracts, all of which do not result in a journal article publication, thus making them more difficult to identify. Studies selected for inclusion in an SR must meet specific predefined criteria, such as the type of research design used, sample selection, length of study, and outcome variables of interest. The identification of RCTs to include in a systematic review is an indirect measure of the availability (or lack thereof) of multiple high-quality studies in a given area. In contrast, a traditional literature or narrative review serves a different purpose in that it deals with a broad range of issues on a given topic rather than answering a specific question in depth. Literature reviews also provide a more subjective assessment in that literature can be selected to support a desired conclusion.[15] A comparison of SRs and literature reviews is illustrated in Table 3-4.

An example of a well-conducted systematic review is demonstrated in the detail of the outline of a Cochrane Systematic Review, as seen in Table 3-5.

Meta-analysis is a statistical process commonly used with systematic reviews. It involves combining the data from multiple individual studies into one analysis. Often smaller RCTs may have rigorous designs but lack

the statistical power to demonstrate a statistically significant effect. When data from these studies are pooled, the sample size and power usually increase. As a result, the combined effect can increase precision of estimates of treatment effects and exposure risks,[13] more so than a SR review in which the data cannot be statistically combined and analyzed.

SECONDARY RESEARCH

Evidence-Based Journals and Article Reviews

Many evidence-based resources have been and are continuing to be developed by evidence-based groups for busy practitioners in order to facilitate the integration of evidence into their clinical decision-making. These include **evidence-based journals** (e.g., *Journal of Evidence Based Dental Practice (JEBDP)*, *Evidence-Based Dentistry (EBD)*, *Evidence-Based Medicine*, *Evidence-Based Nursing*, and *Evidence-Based Healthcare*) and online resources. These journals provide concise and easy-to-read summaries of original and review articles selected from the biomedical literature based on specific inclusion criteria. **Article reviews** of already conducted research often consist of a one- to two-page structured abstract along with an expert commentary highlighting the most relevant and practical information of the study being reviewed.

Evidence-Based Clinical Practice Guidelines

Clinical practice guidelines are a growing source of synthesized information on a specific topic. As defined by the Institute of Medicine, guidelines are "systematically developed statements to assist practitioner and patient decisions about appropriate health care for specific clinical circumstances."[16] The inclusion of scientific evidence within clinical practice guidelines has now become the standard in that guidelines should incorporate the best available scientific evidence. SRs support this process by putting together all that is known about a topic in an objective manner. Examples of clinical practice guidelines include the American Dental Association's clinical recommendations on professionally applied topical fluoride,[17] the American Association of Periodontology's guidelines on the management of patients with periodontal disease,[18] and the American Dental Hygienists' Association's guidelines on polishing procedures.[19]

CONCLUSION

As EBDM becomes standard practice, individuals must be knowledgeable of what constitutes the evidence

---

TABLE 3–4

Cochrane Systematic Review Outline

1. Synopsis
2. Abstract
3. Objectives
4. Criteria for selecting studies:
   - Types of participants
   - Types of intervention
   - Type of outcome measures
   - Types of studies
5. Search strategy
6. Description of studies
7. Methodological quality
8. Results
9. Discussion
10. Reviewers conclusions
11. Acknowledgments
12. Conflicts of interest
13. References
14. Tables and figures

TABLE 3–5

General Characteristics of Systematic Reviews and Traditional Narrative Reviews of the Literature

Characteristic	Systematic Review	Traditional Narrative Review of the Literature
Focus of the review	• Specific problem or patient question; • Narrow focus • Example: Effectiveness of fluoride varnish as compared with topical SnF fluoride in preventing root caries	• Range of issues on a topic • Broad focus • Example: Measures for preventing root surface caries; can include many types of fluorides; may not make comparisons between methods
Who Conducts	*Multidisciplinary Team*	*Individual*
Selection of studies to include	• Preestablished criteria based on validity of study design and specific problem • All studies that meet criteria are included • Systematic bias is minimized based on selection criteria	• Criteria not preestablished or reported in methods. Search on range of issues • May include or exclude studies based on personal bias or support for the hypothesis, if one is stated. • Inherent bias with lack of criteria.
Reported findings	• Search strategy and databases searched • Number of studies that met criteria; number that did not meet and why studies were excluded • Description of study design, subjects, length of trial, state of health/disease, outcome measures	• Literature presented in literature review format and crafted by the individual author • Search strategy, databases, total number of studies pro and con not always identified • Descriptive in nature reporting the outcomes of studies rather than their study designs
Synthesis of selected studies	• Critical analysis of included studies • Determination if results could be statistically combined, and if so, how meta-analysis was conducted	• Reporting of studies that support a procedure or position and those that do not rather than combining data or conducting a statistical analysis
Main results	• Summary of trials, total number of subjects • Definitive statements about the findings in relation to the specified objectives and outcome measures	• Summary of the findings by the author in relation to the purpose of the literature review and specific objectives
Conclusions or comments	• Discussion of the key findings with an interpretation of the results, including potential biases and recommendations for future trials	• Discussion of the key findings with an interpretation of the results, including limitations and recommendations for future trials

and how it is reported. Understanding evidence-based methodology and distinctions between different types of research allows the clinician to better judge the validity and relevance of reported findings. To assist practitioners with this endeavor, new journals devoted to evidence-based practice are being published that alert readers to important advances in a concise and user-friendly manner and the numbers of systematic reviews on clinically relevant topics are increasing. By integrating good science with clinical judgment and patient pref-erences, clinicians enhance their decision-making ability and maximize the potential for successful patient care outcomes.

REFERENCES

1. Greenhalgh T. "Is my practice evidence-based?" Should be answered in qualitative, as well as quantitative terms. *BMJ.* 1996;313:957–958.
2. Hall E. Physical therapists in private practice: information

sources and information needs. *Bull Med Libr Assoc.* 1995;83: 196–201.

3. Gravois S, Bowen D, Fisher W, et al. Dental hygienists' information seeking and computer application behavior. *J Dent Educ.* 1995;59:1027–1033.

4. Curtis K, Weller A. Information-seeking behavior: a survey of health sciences faculty use of indexes and databases. *Bull Med Libr Assoc.* 1993;81:383–392.

5. Horowitz AM, Canto MT, Child WL. Maryland adults' perspectives on oral cancer prevention and early detection. *JADA.* 2002; 133:1061.

6. Giacomini M, Cook D. User's guides to the medical literature: XXIII. Qualitative research in health care A. Are the results of the study valid? *JAMA.* 2000;284:357–362.

7. Giacomini M, Cook D. User's guides to the medical literature: XXIII. Qualitative research in health care B. What are the results and how do they help me care for my patients? *JAMA.* 2000;284:478–482.

8. Albert P, Borkowf C. An introduction to biostatistics: randomization, hypothesis testing and sample size. In: Gallin J, editor. *Principles and Practice of Clinical Research.* San Diego, CA: Academic Press, Elsevier, 2002;163–185.

9. Bossuyt P, Reitsma J, Bruns D, et al. The STARD statement for reporting studies of diagnostic accuracy: explanation and elaboration. *Clin Chem.* 2003;49:7–18.

10. Manolio T. Design and conduct of observational studies and clinical trials. In: Gallin J, editor. *Principles and Practice of Clinical Research.* Academic Press, Elsevier, New York, NY, 2002:187–206.

11. Davis J, Chesney P, Wand P. Toxic shock syndrome: epidemiologic features, recurrence, risk factors, and prevention. *N Engl J Med.* 1980;303:1429.

12. Centers for Disease Control. Pneumocystis pneumonia—Los Angeles. *MMWR Morb Mortal Wkly Rep.* 1981;30:250.

13. Mulrow C. Rationale for systematic reviews. *BMJ.* 1994;309:597–599.

14. SUNY Downstate Medical Center. Guide to research methods, the evidence-based pyramid-systematic reviews and meta-analysis. SUNY Downstate Medical Center Web site. http://library.downstate.edu/EBM2/2700.htm. Accessed September 7, 2006.

15. Sackett D, Haynes R, Guyatt G, et al. *Clinical Epidemiology: A Basic Science for Clinical Medicine.* 2nd ed. Boston: Brown & Company, 1999.

16. Committee on Quality of Health Care in America, IOM. *Crossing the Quality Chasm: A New Health System for the 21st Century.* Washington DC: The National Academy of Sciences, 2000.

17. American Dental Association Council on Scientific Affairs. Professionally applied topical fluoride, evidence-based clinical recommendations. *JADA.* 2006; 137:1151–1159.

18. American Association of Periodontology. Guidelines for the management of patients with periodontal disease. American Association of Periodontology Web site. www.perio.org/resources-products/pdf/management.pdf. Accessed March 31, 2007.

19. American Dental Hygienists Association. ADHA position on polishing procedures. American Dental Hygienists Association Web site. www.adha.org/profissues/polishingpaper.htm. Accessed March 31, 2007.

SUGGESTED ACTIVITIES

At this time, complete the quiz provided here. Then answer the critical thinking questions. Next, complete Exercise 3-1, which asks that you identify whether the described study design is quantitative, qualitative, experimental, nonexperimental primary research or secondary research.

QUIZ

1. Explain why a single research study does not constitute "the evidence."

   _____

   _____

   _____

   _____

   _____

   _____

2. All of the following are considered primary sources of evidence EXCEPT:
   a. RCT
   b. Cohort study
   c. Meta-analysis
   d. Case report

3. Which of the following are considered a secondary source of evidence?
   a. RCT
   b. Cohort study
   c. Meta-analysis
   d. Case report
   e. Case control study

4. Experimental research differs from nonexperimental research in that it:
   a. Makes observations without intervening
   b. Focuses retrospectively
   c. Studies rare diseases
   d. Tests cause and effect
   e. Has no control group

5. Match the study design with its characteristic:

   Study Design   Characteristic

   a. Case control   _____ Prospective without any intervention
   b. Cohort study   _____ Tests cause and effect
   c. RCT   _____ Synthesis of two or more studies
   d. Case report   _____ No control group
   e. Systematic review   _____ Single patient observation

6. Characteristics of experimental research include:
   a. Randomizing subjects to treatment and control groups
   b. Randomly allocating treatments
   c. Ability to blind studies
   d. Retrospective analysis
   e. a, b, and c
   f. All of the above

7. Characteristics of nonexperimental research include:
   a. Making observations between exposures and diseases
   b. Ability to conduct studies prospectively
   c. Ability to conduct studies retrospectively
   d. Reports of a single case
   e. a, b, and c
   f. All of the above

8. Match the type of research (A or B) with the characteristics list below.
   A. Qualitative research   or   B. Quantitative research

   _____ Tests a hypothesis

   _____ Provides explanations

   _____ Data are collected via fieldwork

   _____ Analysis occurs after all data are collected

   _____ Tests cause and effects

   _____ Examines associations between exposure and risk factor

   _____ Data reported in narrative terms

   _____ Can generate hypotheses

CRITICAL THINKING QUESTIONS

1. Discuss how quantitative and qualitative research are complementary and provide an example of a study related to patient problems that would include both types of studies. (Example: how often patients floss [quantitative study] and what barriers do they encounter that prevents them from flossing every day [qualitative study]).

   _____

   _____

   _____

   _____

   _____

2. Explain why an RCT is not always the appropriate research design to use.

   _____

   _____

   _____

   _____

   _____

3. Provide an example of when you would first conduct a traditional literature search before looking for a systematic review or meta-analysis.

   _____

   _____

   _____

   _____

   _____

EXERCISE 3-1

Identify whether the described study design is quantitative, qualitative, experimental, nonexperimental, primary research, or secondary research. Please check all that apply.

Check all that apply:

1. Randomly assigned subjects, randomly assigned treatments, experimental and control groups

- ☐ Quantitative
- ☐ Qualitative
- ☐ Experimental
- ☐ Nonexperimental
- ☐ Primary research
- ☐ Secondary research

2. Systematic statement to assist decision-making about care for specific circumstances

- ☐ Quantitative
- ☐ Qualitative
- ☐ Experimental
- ☐ Nonexperimental
- ☐ Primary research
- ☐ Secondary research

3. Compilation of data from multiple studies selected using explicit criteria that answers a specific question

- ☐ Quantitative
- ☐ Qualitative
- ☐ Experimental
- ☐ Nonexperimental
- ☐ Primary research
- ☐ Secondary research

4. Observes associations between risk factors and the development of a disease

- ☐ Quantitative
- ☐ Qualitative
- ☐ Experimental
- ☐ Nonexperimental
- ☐ Primary research
- ☐ Secondary research

5. Reports the treatment of a single patient or several patients with the same condition

- ☐ Quantitative
- ☐ Qualitative
- ☐ Experimental
- ☐ Nonexperimental
- ☐ Primary research
- ☐ Secondary research

6. A retrospective study that observes possible associations between a disease and one or more hypothesized risk factors

- ☐ Quantitative
- ☐ Qualitative
- ☐ Experimental
- ☐ Nonexperimental
- ☐ Primary research
- ☐ Secondary research

7. Describes real experiences of individuals as interpreted by the researcher

- ☐ Quantitative
- ☐ Qualitative
- ☐ Experimental
- ☐ Nonexperimental
- ☐ Primary research
- ☐ Secondary research

NOTES

CHAPTER 4

Levels of Evidence

PURPOSE

Evidence-based decision making is about solving clinical problems and involves two fundamental principles: 1) evidence alone is never sufficient to make a clinical decision, and 2) a hierarchy of evidence exists to guide clinical decision making.[1] The purpose of this section is to discuss the hierarchy, or levels of evidence, which are based on the notion of causation and the need to control bias.[2] The focus will be on quantitative research and questions related to therapy/prevention, harm/etiology/causation, prognosis, and diagnosis.

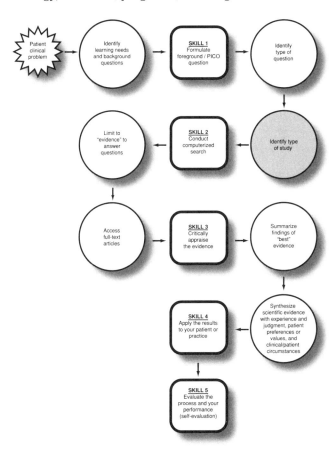

OBJECTIVES

After completing this chapter, readers will be able to:

1. Identify the levels of evidence.
2. Identify the type of study most appropriate to answer questions related to therapy/prevention, diagnosis, harm/etiology/causation, and prognosis.

3. Explain how each research study design contributes to a continuum of knowledge.

SUGGESTED ACTIVITIES

Quiz
Critical Thinking Questions
Exercise 4-1
Exercise 4-2

LEVELS OF EVIDENCE

Evidence-based medicine groups have defined what constitutes strong evidence as it relates to human beings as opposed to animal and laboratory studies.[2,3] The hierarchy of evidence is based on the notion of causation and the need to control bias.[4] **Levels of evidence** are based on research study designs and they rank the validity of evidence, allowing the user to put confidence in the results. For example, a randomized controlled trial (RCT) provides stronger evidence than a cohort or case control study when testing a therapy (Fig. 4-1).

Although each level may contribute to the total body of knowledge, . . . "not all levels are equally useful for making patient care decisions."[5] As one progresses up the levels, the number of studies and, correspondingly, the amount of available literature decreases, while at the same time their relevance to answering clinical questions increases. Knowing which type of research study provides the strongest level of evidence for the question being asked is important in conducting an evidence-based search of the literature.

Levels of evidence and grades of recommendations were initially developed by Fletcher and Sackett in 1979 for the Canadian Task Force on the Periodic Health Examination. The levels ranking the validity of preventive procedures were then tied to grades of recommendations.[3] Since that time, levels of evidence and grades of recommendations, or types of evidence and their ratings, have been adapted and refined by different health care groups using a variety of formats.[2,6] Although different evaluation and grading systems are used, these models for categorizing studies are helpful in determining the level of evidence available for answering clinically related questions and serve as a basis for identifying the strength of the evidence as being strong, moderate,

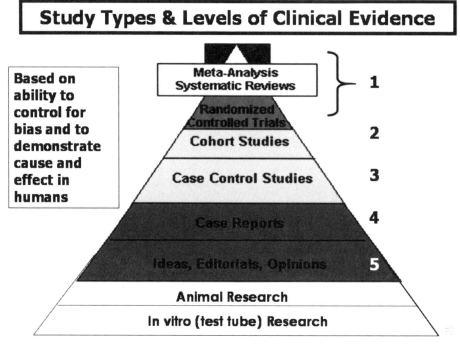

FIGURE 4–1 Levels of clinical evidence for therapy/prevention and etiology/harm. Modified Evidence Pyramid. Copyright permission granted by SUNY Downstate Medical Center, Medical Research Library at Brooklyn, http://library.downstate.edu/EBM2/2100.htm

limited, or missing evidence related to areas of practice (Table 4-1).

RELATIONSHIP BETWEEN THE TYPE OF QUESTION AND TYPE OF STUDY

Evidence is judged on its rigor of methodology and the level of evidence is directly related to the type of question asked, such as those derived from issues of therapy/prevention, diagnosis, etiology, and prognosis. For example, the highest level of evidence associated with questions about therapy or prevention will be from systematic reviews of RCT studies (Table 4-2) because the objective of these studies is to test interventions demonstrating cause and effect and to select treatments that improve the condition/disease and avoid adverse events.[1] However, the highest level of evidence associated with questions about prognosis will be from systematic reviews of inception cohort studies[2] (Table 4-2) because

TABLE 4–1

Levels of Evidence, Strength, and Grade of Recommendation

Level of Evidence	Strength	Grade of Rx
Level 1 studies	Strong	A
Level 2 or 3 studies OR extrapolations* from level 1 studies	Moderate	B
Level 4 studies OR extrapolations from level 2 or 3 studies	Limited/weak	C
Level 5 evidence OR troublingly inconsistent or inconclusive studies of any level	Incomplete/ insufficient	D

Adapted from the Centre for Evidence-Based Medicine, www.cebm.net/levels_of_evidence.asp#levels.
*"Extrapolations" are where data are used in a situation that has potentially clinically important differences than the original study situation.

TABLE 4-2

Type of Question Related to Levels of Evidence and Study Methodology

Type of Question	Type of Study or Methodology of Choice[2]	Question Focus[9,10]	Why Study?[1,9,10]	Example Questions
Therapy/ prevention	Meta-analysis or systematic review of RCTs Single randomized controlled trial SR of cohort studies	Study effect of therapy or test on real patients; allows for comparison between intervention group and control groups for a particular condition. Largest volume of EB literature	To select treatments, if any, that do more good than harm (improve function, avoid adverse events) that are worth the effort and cost	Do sealed permanent first molars need less restorative treatment than unsealed permanent first molars?
Diagnosis	Meta-analysis or SR of controlled trials (prospective cohort study) Single controlled trial (Prospective—compare tests with a reference or "gold" standard test)	Measures reliability of a particular diagnostic measure/test for a disease against the "gold standard" diagnostic measure for the same disease. Sensitivity and specificity of the measures are compared.	To select and interpret diagnostic methods or tests. To determine the degree to which a test is reliable and useful; establish the power of an intervention to differentiate between those with and without a target condition or disease.	How reliable is the D-N saliva test as compared with current caries activity for predicting future caries activity?
Etiology, causation, harm	Meta-analysis or SR of RCTs Single RCT SR of cohort studies Single cohort study (prospective data collection with formal control group)	Compares a group exposed to a particular agent with an unexposed group. Important for understanding prevention and control of disease.	To identify causes of a disease or condition including iatrogenic forms. To determine relationships between risk factors, potentially harmful agents, and possible causes of a disease or condition.	Does smoking influence vertical alveolar bone loss?
Prognosis	Meta-analysis or SR of inception cohort studies (follow patients from when disease 1st becomes clinically manifest) Cohort study	Follows progression of a group with particular disease and compares with a group without the disease. Groups must be as similar as possible and must have good follow-up >80% of each group.	To estimate clinical course or progression of a disease or condition over time and anticipate likely complications (and prevent them).	What patient and implant characteristics influence the survival of dental implants?

SR: systematic review; RCT: randomized controlled study; EB: evidence-based; D-N:.

the objective of these studies is to estimate the future course of a patient's disease over time and to anticipate likely complications. **Inception cohort studies** are those in which the cohort of subjects are all initially free of the outcome of interest and are followed until the oc-currence of either a major study end point or end of the study.[2]

For studies related to diagnosis, the levels of evidence are related to the accuracy of the diagnostic test in terms of its sensitivity and specificity. *Sensitivity* refers to the proportion of people with disease who have a positive test.[7] In other words, the diagnostic test is able to accurately identify those who actually have the disease as having the disease. *Specificity* is the proportion of people free of a disease who have a negative test; that is, the ability of the test to correctly identify those who do not have a disease as not having the disease.[8] For studies related to diagnosis, the highest level is a systematic review of Level 1 diagnostic studies, which means that the following conditions are met when a new diagnostic test is being considered.[2]

1. Subjects/participants receive *both* the new diagnostic test and the currently accepted reference or gold standard test.
2. A range of participants is included: those who are disease free, have moderate disease, and have severe disease so that the new diagnostic test can be evaluated for a broad scope of conditions.
3. Examiners are not aware of which test was used or the disease status of the subjects.
4. Results (sensitivity and specificity) are then compared to see if the new test is as accurate as the currently accepted reference or gold standard test.

This procedure is considered a controlled trial, but not a randomized controlled trial because subjects receive both the new diagnostic test and the gold standard test. Therefore the highest level of evidence is a systematic review of controlled trials (Table 4-2) because the purpose is to determine the degree to which a test is reliable and useful.

An important concept to recognize is that, at all levels, having a systematic review provides stronger evidence than a single study. Table 4-2 illustrates this and also demonstrates this concept while identifying the focus and purpose of the studies related to therapy/prevention, diagnosis, etiology, causation and harm, and prognosis.

Correctly identifying the type of study to answer the question is an important skill to develop to access the appropriate evidence when searching the health care literature. For example, identifying the best strategy for managing an endodontic lesion is a treatment question. Ideally, a meta-analysis or systematic review of RCTs would be available that synthesized the research on the endodontic treatment being considered. If these were not available, then the next best evidence would be from a well-conducted individual RCT. However, when the focus of the question is on long-term outcomes of treatment, then it is a question of prognosis. In this case, the highest level of evidence would be provided by a systematic review of inception cohort studies, which are studies that follow patients from when a disease or condition first manifests itself clinically. And again, if a systematic review was not available, the next highest level would be an individual inception cohort study, and so on down the hierarchy (Table 4-2).

LEVELS OF EVIDENCE PROVIDE A CONTINUUM OF KNOWLEDGE—WATER FLUORIDATION EXAMPLE

It is important to recognize that evidence may be used in all of its forms. Each of the primary research study designs contributes to a continuum of knowledge development and validation (Table 4-3). A classic example of this continuum in oral health is the discovery of water fluoridation and its relationship to mottled enamel and caries incidence. Dr. Frederick S. McKay made the first **case report** in 1901 noting that many of his patients in Colorado Springs, CO, had permanently stained teeth.[11] Later, with the help of Dr. G.V. Black in 1909, this condition was termed *mottled enamel*. McKay **hypothesized** that the cause was linked to the drinking water, as did Dr. John Eager in his observations of US-bound Italian emigrants from Naples, Italy. Eager noted that when Naples changed its drinking water source, the incidence of stained teeth among infants greatly diminished.[11] Dr. McKay later noted in 1925 that children who lived in areas where mottled enamel was prevalent also had fewer caries.

McKay continued his investigations and advocated for testing water supplies in communities where mottled enamel disfigured the teeth of children. These **clinical observations led to experimental animal studies,**[12] and later to the **cohort study** examining the relationship between fluoride in water supplies and mottled enamel by Dr. H. Trendley Dean of the US Public Health Service. Dean also focused on the link between mottled enamel and the incidence of dental caries and began investigating the effectiveness and safety of fluoridated water. Surveys of school children revealed that those in communities with fluoride had fewer caries than those children living in communities with little fluoride in the water.

By quantifying fluoride levels in drinking water, 1 ppm was identified as a safe level that did not cause mottling or have toxic effects. These clinical observations and survey findings were then tested using a **prospective community-based controlled clinical trial**, the Grand Rapids fluoridation project, initiated in 1945. This clinical trial confirmed that 1 ppm fluoride significantly lowered the incidence of dental caries without mottled enamel or other side effects. Thus a case report of clinical observations, one of the lowest levels of evidence, led to the development of hypotheses that were tested and validated through more rigorously designed scientific studies and appropriately designed controlled clinical trials.

TABLE 4-3

Continuum of Knowledge Derived from Different Study Designs

Study Design	Objectives	Methods	Benefits	Disadvantages
Experimental, randomized, controlled trial (prospective)	Test interventions demonstrating cause and effect; standard for evaluating therapeutic efficacy	Experimental group and control group; randomization of subjects and treatments; blinding of subjects and investigators	Provides strongest evidence for causality; minimizes bias via randomization and blinding; internal and external validity	Cost, time, and ethical considerations
Nonexperimental cohort study (prospective)	Observe association about exposure or risk factor and subsequent development of disease/condition; determine diagnosis and etiology of disease	Exposure group compared to nonexposure group; prospective— subjects do not have the disease/condition of interest; measures made before disease development	Ability to establish temporal sequence; ability to control and monitor data collection and measure variables accurately. Useful when disease/condition occurs frequently.	Time to develop disease or condition, cost of follow-up and losing subjects over time. Difficult to establish causation.
Case control (retrospective)	Observations about possible associations between disease and one or more hypothesized risk factors. Determine etiology of disease.	Retrospective— subjects already have disease or condition and are compared with representative group of disease-free persons— controls from the same population.	Useful in studying potential etiologies of rare diseases or diseases with long lag periods between exposure and outcome; cost and when ethical reasons do not allow randomized RCTs controlled trials.	Looks back—recall bias and incomplete sources for information; identification of comparison group and case selection. Difficult to establish causation.
Case series (several similar cases) or case report (single case)	Documentation of unique or unusual condition with clinical characteristics.	Present as complete a picture of clinical data, potential exposures, or causal factors. Detailed to permit recognition of similar cases by others.	Useful in forming hypotheses and describing clinical experiences; clues for further research; easy and inexpensive.	No statistical validity. Bias in selection of patients; lacks control so not able to generalize.

LEVELS OF EVIDENCE FOR GAIL

At this time, it is important to consider the levels of evidence that are pertinent for Gail. In doing so, Part B of the evidence-based decision-making worksheet is completed. Because the question for Gail is one of therapy, it was completed as shown in Figure 4-2.

EBDM Worksheet PART B

Understanding the Publication Type So That Appropriate Studies Can Be Identified

1. Type of study (publication type) to include in the search (check all that apply, then number from highest [1] to lowest level of evidence).

☑ __1__ Meta-analysis	☑ __2__ Systematic review	☑ __3__ Randomized controlled trial
☑ __4__ Clinical trial	☑ __5__ Practice guideline	☐ _____ Review
☐ _____ Cohort study	☐ _____ Case control study	☐ _____ Case series or case report
☐ _____ Editorials, letters, opinions	☐ _____ Animal research	☐ _____ In vitro/lab research

---

FIGURE 4–2 Levels of Evidence for Gail

CONCLUSION

A hierarchy of evidence exists to guide clinical decision making. As evidence-based decision-making becomes standard practice, knowing the levels of evidence helps the practitioner determine the strength of the evidence, whether provided by a systematic review or individual study. In turn, understanding research design and distinctions between different types of study methods, such as an RCT and a cohort study, and the type of question being answered allows the clinician to better judge the validity and relevance of reported findings.

REFERENCES

1. Evidence-based Medicine Working Group. *Users' Guides to the Medical Literature, A Manual for EB Clinical Practice.* Chicago: AMA Press, 2002.
2. Phillips B, Ball C, Sackett D, et al. Levels of evidence and grades of recommendations. 2001. Centre for Evidence-Based Medicine Web site. http://www.cebm.net/levels_of_evidence.asp. Accessed March 18, 2007.
3. Canadian Task Force on the Periodic Health Examination. The periodic health examination. *CMAJ.* 1979;121:1193–1254.
4. Long A, Harrison S. The balance of evidence. Evidence-based decision making. *Health Serv J.* 1995;6(Glaxo Welcome Suppl):1–2.
5. McKibbon A, Eady A, Marks S. *PDQ, Evidence-Based Principles and Practice.* Hamilton, Ontario: B.C. Decker Inc., 1999.
6. Health Evidence Bulletins: Wales. Oral cancer evidence. Health Evidence Bulletins: Wales Web site. http://hebw.uwcm.ac.uk/oralhealth/chapter4.html#Oral%20Cancer. Accessed March 18, 2007.
7. Centre for Evidence-Based Medicine. SpPins and SnNouts. Centre for Evidence-Based Medicine Web site. www.cebm.net/sppins_snnouts.asp. Accessed March 18, 2007.
8. Centre for Evidence-Based Medicine. Levels of evidence and grades of recommendations. Centre for Evidence-Based Medicine Web site. http://www.cebm.net/levels_of_evidence.asp. Accessed March 18, 2007.
9. Haynes R, Wilczynski N, McKibbon A, et al. Developing optimal search strategies for detecting clinically sound studies in MEDLINE. *J Am Med Inform Assoc.* 1994;1:447–458.
10. Duke University Medical Center Library, Health Sciences Library University of North Carolina at Chapel Hill. Introduction to evidence-based medicine, the well-built clinical question. Duke University Medical Center Library and Health Sciences Library University of North Carolina at Chapel Hill Web site. http://www.hsl.unc.edu/Services/Tutorials/EBM/index.htm. Accessed March 18, 2007.
11. Harris R. *Dental Science in a New Age: A History of the National Institute of Dental Research.* Rockville, MD: Montrose Press, 1989.
12. Smith M, Lantz E, Smith H. Cause of mottled enamel, defect of human teeth. Science. 1931;74:244. Univ Ariz Agr Exp Sta Tech Bull.

SUGGESTED ACTIVITIES

At this time, complete the quiz provided here. Then answer the critical thinking questions.

QUIZ

1. Put the levels of evidence in order of their ability to demonstrate causality and limit bias with A = highest ability and E = lowest ability.

   _____ Case control study

   _____ Cohort study

   _____ Systematic review

   _____ Randomized controlled trial

   _____ Case report

2. Systematic reviews provide a higher level of evidence than a single study.
   A. True
   B. False

3. As you progress up the levels of evidence, the amount of available literature also increases.
   A. True
   B. False

4. As you progress up the levels of evidence, the literature becomes more relevant for answering clinical questions.
   A. True
   B. False

5. Match the following characteristics with the type of question.
   A. Therapy/prevention
   B. Diagnosis
   C. Etiology/harm
   D. Prognosis

   _____ Compares a group exposed to a particular risk with an unexposed group

   _____ Controlled trial

   _____ Comparison between intervention group and control groups

   _____ Inception cohort study

   _____ Systematic review of RCTs

   _____ Follows progression of a group with particular condition and compares with a group without the condition

   _____ Measures reliability of a particular test for a disease against the "gold standard"

   _____ Systematic review of cohort studies

CRITICAL THINKING QUESTIONS

1. Explain why evidence alone is never sufficient to make a clinical decision.

_____

_____

_____

_____

_____

_____

_____

_____

_____

2. Discuss why a controlled trial is used when testing a new diagnostic test.

_____

_____

_____

_____

_____

_____

_____

_____

_____

3. Explain how all types of research may contribute to a continuum of knowledge.

_____

_____

_____

_____

_____

_____

_____

_____

EXERCISE 4-1

This exercise focuses on having you identify the types of studies that will provide the highest level of evidence for that question and then list them in order. For each question, list the type of study to include in the search in order from highest to lowest level of evidence, with 1 being the highest. If you need to review, the type of question was discussed in Chapter 2 and completed in Exercise 2-1. For example, for a therapy question, meta-analysis, systematic review, RCT, and clinical trial may be the types of studies you would identify. Then you would list them in order beginning with the type of study that provides the highest level of evidence.

Type of study to include in the search (use all that apply)

Meta-analysis of _____	Systematic review of _____	Randomized controlled trial
Clinical trial	Controlled trial	Review
Cohort study	Case control study	Case series or case report
Editorials, letters, opinions	Animal research	In vitro/lab research

Example
For adults with overlapping central incisors, will Invisalign as compared to orthodontic braces correctly align the incisors in shorter time period, at less cost?

1. Meta-analysis of RCTs
2. Systematic review of RCTs
3. Individual RCT
4. Systematic review of cohort studies
5. Individual cohort study

For dentists/dental hygienists with neck and shoulder pain, will correct posture and use of magnification and illumination reduce the pain?

1.
2.
3.
4.
5.

For parents with infants, will chewing xylitol gum result in suppression of mutans streptococci and transmission of MS to their children?

1.
2.
3.
4.
5.

For children and adolescents, will fluoride varnish as compared to a fluoride rinse prevent dental caries?

1.
2.
3.
4.
5.

For a patient with amalgam restorations, will leaving the amalgam restorations intact as compared to replacing them with composite or a crown, result in no adverse general or oral health effects?

1.
2.
3.
4.
5.

For patients with a suspicious lesion, is toluidine blue, an adjunctive diagnostic aid, compared to the Oral CDx brush biopsy technique more accurate as a screening device in detecting oral cancer?

1.
2.
3.
4.
5.

EXERCISE 4-2

This exercise completes Part B of the EBDM worksheet, which focuses on having you identify the types of studies that will provide the highest level of evidence for each of the 5 case scenarios introduced in Chapter 2. Identify the appropriate type of study according to the type of question being asked. Number them from highest to lowest level of evidence, with 1 being the highest. Refer to the case scenarios and Exercise 2-2 if clarification is needed.

Morty

Mr. Morty Kramer, a 55-year-old man, has been using unwaxed floss his whole life and flosses frequently. At his last dental appointment, he was treated by a new hygienist, who told him that he needed to change to using a waxed floss because it is more effective in removing plaque. Morty is happy with his current oral hygiene regimen and asks if he really needs to change.

Trevor

Trevor is a 27-year-old bartender who has used chewing tobacco for 13 years. He is a frequent user who chews almost 5 hours a day. He has just learned from his oral health care provider that he has developed precancerous lesions in the vestibular area where he holds the tobacco plug. This new information has motivated him to quit. Trevor knows he can't quit by willpower alone because he has tried in the past. He wants to know if a non-nicotine aid in tobacco cessation is helpful in this endeavor or if a nicotine patch is better in helping users permanently quit. He would like to know if behavioral therapy/counseling might help.

Dr. Bailer

Dr. Bailer recently graduated from dental school and is building a new dental practice. As he designs his building, he is trying to decide whether to purchase digital radiograph equipment or to use traditional radiography. He is interested in knowing the most accurate method for caries detection.

Jennifer

Your morning patient, Mrs. Jennifer Morris, comes to you distressed because of an article she read on the Internet about the dangers of mercury in her amalgam restorations. She is worried that her seven amalgam fillings are poisoning her. She is very concerned not only for her own health but for her two young daughters that also have amalgam restorations. Jennifer doesn't want to replace her fillings if it isn't necessary, but needs proof that she and her children are going to be healthy.

To reassure your patient, you give her advice based on your clinical experience and judgment; however, she still seems very upset and troubled. You inform her that you will do a thorough search of the current scientific literature and get back to her with your findings. She seems more relaxed with this thought and leaves eager to hear from you soon.

Sam

Sam is a 49-year-old man with moderate periodontitis, who was recently diagnosed with type 2 diabetes mellitus. Sam's glycosylated hemoglobin (HbA1) is 12%, which places him in the category of poorly controlled diabetes. Sam is worried that his diabetes will increase his chance of losing his teeth. He wants to know the effect and impact diabetes now has on his oral health.

EBDM Worksheet PART B

Understanding the Publication Type So That Appropriate Studies Can Be Identified

1. Type of study (publication type) to include in the search (check all that apply, then number from highest [1] to lowest level of evidence).

☐ _____ Meta-analysis   ☐ _____ Systematic review   ☐ _____ Randomized controlled trial

☐ _____ Clinical trial   ☐ _____ Practice guideline   ☐ _____ Review

☐ _____ Cohort study   ☐ _____ Case control study   ☐ _____ Case series or case report

☐ _____ Editorials, letters, opinions   ☐ _____ Animal research   ☐ _____ In vitro/lab research

CHAPTER 5

Finding the Evidence: Using PICO to Guide the Search

SKILL 2

Conducting a Computerized Search with Maximum Efficiency for Finding the Best External Evidence with Which to Answer the Question.

PURPOSE

The purpose of this section is to focus on strategies to integrate the second step of the evidence-based decision-making (EBDM) approach, the computerized search, into practice. It will provide an overview of the main biomedical databases including, The Cochrane Library (Systematic Reviews and Abstracts), CINAHL, and MEDLINE and will demonstrate how to find valid evidence to answer PICO questions using PubMed, which provides free access to the MEDLINE database. Steps involved in structuring and conducting the search will be outlined and case scenarios will demonstrate the application of the skills involved. It may be helpful to complete the PubMed tutorial at www.pubmed.gov before reading this chapter. Also, using PubMed in conjunction with reading each step of the searching process related to the Gail case later in this section will aid in the understanding of the concepts outlined in this section.

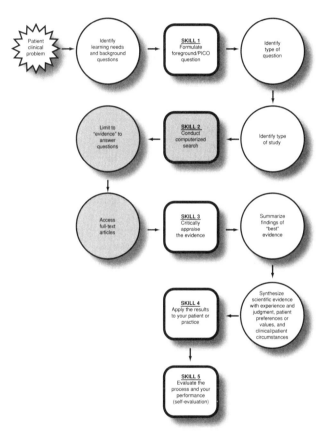

OBJECTIVES

After completing this chapter, readers will be able to:

1. Identify at least two databases in which secondary and primary research can be found.
2. Explain the type of research that can be found using PubMed, CINAHL, and the Cochrane Library databases (Cochrane Database of Systematic Reviews, DARE, The Cochrane Controlled Trials Register).
3. Describe how PubMed is structured and discuss the key searching components (i.e., medical subject headings [MeSH] terms, Boolean Operators, History, and Limits).
4. Find MeSH terms for a PICO question using the PubMed MeSH browser.
5. Given a PICO question or clinical topic, effectively use PubMed to find evidence to answer a PICO question using the key functions of PubMed including: MeSH, Boolean Operators, Search History, Limits, and Clinical Queries.

SUGGESTED ACTIVITIES

Quiz
Critical Thinking Questions
Exercise 5-1

After a good clinical question has been formulated using the PICO process, the second step in using EBDM is to conduct a computerized search to find the best external evidence for answering the question. This type of search requires a shift in thinking. Often, especially now with fast web-based search engines, health professionals look for "something" on a topic, a quick answer, or for "everything." Finding relevant evidence requires conducting a very focused search of the peer-reviewed professional literature based on the appropriate research methodology.

PICO PROVIDES THE FOUNDATION FOR THE SEARCH

The PICO question provides the foundation for the search terms used in the database. By combining the patient problem or description with the intervention, comparison, and/or outcome, one can quickly pinpoint a set of citations that will potentially provide an answer to the question being posed. Online databases and software enable quick access to the literature, making it easier to locate relevant clinical evidence. Knowing how databases filter information and having an understanding of how to use PICO facilitates a search of the literature with maximum efficiency.

FINDING THE EVIDENCE

Secondary Research

Secondary research, which includes the meta-analysis, systematic reviews, and clinical practice guidelines, evidence-based journals, and article reviews, was discussed in Chapter 3. Now we will discuss how these studies can be accessed online.

The Cochrane Collaboration, an international, volunteer, nonprofit organization comprising academics, clinicians, researchers, industry representatives, and journal editors, is a valuable resource for clinicians. It was established in 1992 to facilitate conducting systematic reviews of randomized controlled trials across all areas of health care.[1] Today there are more than 50 specialist review groups in more than 13 countries covering each area within health care, including oral health, that provide peer-reviewed systematic reviews meeting international standards.[2] The results of their work are housed in the Cochrane Library, which contains:

1. The Cochrane Database of Systematic Reviews (COCH): includes the full text of the regularly updated systematic reviews of the effects of health care prepared by The Cochrane Collaboration. The reviews are presented in two types:
   Complete reviews—regularly updated Cochrane Reviews, prepared and maintained by collaborative review groups
   Protocols—protocols for reviews currently being prepared (all include an expected date of completion). Protocols are the background, objectives, and methods of reviews in preparation.
2. Database of Abstracts of Reviews of Effectiveness (DARE): a collection of structured literature abstracts, which have been critically appraised by reviewers at

the British National Health Service (NHS) Center for Reviews and Dissemination at the University of York.
3. The Cochrane Controlled Trials Register (CCTR): a bibliography of controlled trials identified by contributors to the Cochrane Collaboration and others as part of an international effort to hand search the world's journals and create an unbiased source of data for systematic reviews.[2]

Primary Research

The first step of finding valid evidence is knowing where to look. We have already discussed some of the sources for secondary research. There are many databases that contain both primary research studies and secondary sources such as systematic reviews. Knowing where to find the research is important so that key articles and evidence are accessed from the search.

This workbook will be highlighting MEDLINE/PubMed as the main database for dentistry and dental hygiene. PubMed is used in this section because it is the free access to MEDLINE. Many schools subscribe to MEDLINE through OVID, which, for some, is easier to use and provides access to many full-text articles. **OVID** is an information search platform that includes Ovid Gateway and SilverPlatter that allows users to access electronic citations, including journals, books, and databases—such as CINAHL and MEDLINE, with tools to browse, search, retrieve, and analyze critical information. However, OVID is subscription-based and many practitioners do not have access to it after graduation. Therefore, for purposes of accessibility, PubMed, the free access to MEDLINE, will be used to search for scientific evidence in this workbook.

The CINAHL Database

CINAHL, The Cumulative Index to Nursing and Allied Health, contains scientific evidence related to dentistry and dental hygiene; however, it also is a subscription based database. If your school has access to OVID, CINAHL may be one of the included databases to which the school subscribes. This database provides access to journals related to nursing and other allied health fields, including dental hygiene.[3]

Although we are not providing examples of how to search CINAHL, it is important to point out the main differences from MEDLINE. First, CINAHL has more than 2,400 subject headings that are unique to CINAHL that can be used to search the literature. These were developed to reflect the language used by nursing and allied health professionals. Second, CINAHL has specific interest categories to search for relevant literature, such as women's or men's health, patient safety, and dental care. Familiarizing yourself with these features enables a more accurate search of the literature contained in this database.[4,5]

TABLE 5-1

Web Sites of Research Sources

Name	URL
The Cochrane Database of Systematic Reviews	www.cochrane.org/reviews/index.htm
DARE (Database of Abstracts of Reviews of Effectiveness)	www.cochrane.org/reviews/index.htm or www.crd.york.ac.uk/crdweb
The Cochrane Controlled Trials Register	www.cochrane.org/reviews/index.htm
PubMed, Free access to MEDLINE, National Library of Medicine	www.pubmed.gov/
CINAHL	www.cinahl.com/

MEDLINE Database

MEDLINE is the bibliographic database of the National Library of Medicine (NLM). It contains bibliographic citations and author abstracts that cover the fields of medicine, nursing, dentistry, and veterinary medicine. As of 2007, MEDLINE contains citations from more than 5,000 biomedical journals published in the United States and 80 other countries. It comprises more than 15 million citations starting from the mid-1950s. Although coverage is worldwide, most sources are written in English or have English abstracts.[5]

PubMed

PubMed is an online database that provides free access to citations from biomedical literature, including MEDLINE and access and links to other molecular biology resources. If publishers have a Web site that offers their journals and full-text articles online, PubMed provides links to that site as well as to biologic resources, consumer health information, research tools, and more; however, there may be a charge to access the full text or information (Table 5-1).[5]

HOW TO SEARCH: KEY FEATURES OF PUBMED

Each database has its own set of searching tips that are helpful when looking for evidence to answer the question. Our focus will be the steps involved in conducting a PubMed search using a search strategy to retrieve relevant evidence to answer a PICO question.

Tutorial

PubMed has an online tutorial that walks through all the steps of a search and explains each PubMed feature and tool so that users understand the language, or how information on the database is indexed (www.pubmed.gov/). How the database is searched, how citations can be limited to the most relevant articles, and how search terms can be combined is thoroughly explained in the tutorial. Some of the features outlined in the tutorial will be introduced here.

MeSH

The NLM uses a controlled vocabulary of biomedical terms to index articles, catalog books and other holdings, and facilitate searching within MEDLINE. **Medical subject headings (MeSH)** describe the subject of each journal article in the database. MeSH terms provide a consistent way of retrieving information that uses different terminology for the same concept. MeSH terms are indexed hierarchically by category, with more specific terms arranged beneath broader terms.[6] PubMed has a MeSH browser, www.nlm.nih.gov/mesh/MBrowser.html, that aids in the identification of the appropriate terms for how articles are indexed on a specific topic (Fig. 5-1).[7]

By opening this browser, one can enter a text word and it will show the MEDLINE MeSH term descriptor and how the term is structured in the hierarchical "MeSH tree." When typing the term "dry mouth" into the browser, it provides the option to select either xerostomia or Mouth Dryness. By selecting either of these, the MeSH Descriptor data for xerostomia is displayed (Fig. 5-2).

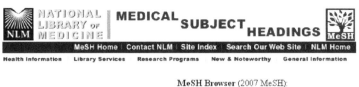

MeSH Browser (2007 MeSH):
The files are updated every week on Sunday
Go to 2006 MeSH

Enter term or the beginning of any root fragments: or   [Navigate from tree top]

[   ]

Search for these record types: ○ **Search in these fields of chemicals:**

○ Main Headings   ☐ Heading Mapped To (HM) (Supplementary List)

○ Qualifiers   ☐ Indexing Information (II) (Supplementary List)

○ Supplementary Concepts   ☐ Pharmacological Action (PA)

⊙ All of the Above   ☐ CAS Registry/EC Number (RN)

○ Search as MeSH Unique ID   ☐ Related CAS Registry Number (RR)

○ Search as text words in Annotation & Scope Note

[Find Exact Term]   [Find Terms with ALL Fragments]   [Find Terms with ANY Fragment]

MeSH
vocabulary
suggestions

About MeSH Browser | MeSH Home Page | Questions or Comments
NLM Classification, the scheme used to categorize and organize books, audiovisuals, and similar materials.

FIGURE 5–1   MeSH browser.

National Library of Medicine - Medical Subject Headings

2007 MeSH

MeSH Descriptor Data

Return to Entry Page

MeSH Heading	Xerostomia
Tree Number	C07.465.815.929
Annotation	decreased saliva flow
Scope Note	Decreased salivary flow.
Entry Term	Asialia
Entry Term	Hyposalivation
Entry Term	Mouth Dryness
Allowable Qualifiers	BL CF CI CL CN CO DH DI DT EC EH EM EN EP ET GE HI IM ME MI MO NU PA PC PP PS PX RA RH RI RT SU TH UR US VE VI
Unique ID	D014987

FIGURE 5–2   MeSH descriptor data for xerostomia.

Here we see that the MeSH term "xerostomia" is annotated and scope noted as "Decreased salivary flow." By clicking on the Tree Number, it shows how the term is indexed by the MeSH Tree Structures under Stomatognathic Diseases, Mouth Diseases, Salivary Gland Diseases (Fig. 5-3). Knowing how the term is indexed is especially helpful if the search does not retrieve enough articles. This provides terminology to broaden the search to the higher levels of the MeSH tree.

MeSH Tree Structures

Stomatognathic Diseases [C07]
  Mouth Diseases [C07.465]
    Salivary Gland Diseases [C07.465.815]
                    Mikulicz' Disease [C07.465.815.355]
                    Parotid Diseases [C07.465.815.470] +
                    Salivary Duct Calculi [C07.465.815.525]
                    Salivary Gland Calculi [C07.465.815.594]
                    Salivary Gland Fistula [C07.465.815.655]
                    Salivary Gland Neoplasms [C07.465.815.718] +
                    Sialadenitis [C07.465.815.793] +
                    Sialometaplasia, Necrotizing [C07.465.815.802]
                    Sialorrhea [C07.465.815.815]
                    Submandibular Gland Diseases [C07.465.815.882] +
                ➤ Xerostomia [C07.465.815.929]
                        Sjogren's Syndrome [C07.465.815.929.669]

FIGURE 5–3   MeSH tree structures for xerostomia.

Clinical and Special Queries

Other valuable tools for conducting an evidence-based search are the Clinical Queries and Special Queries features. The clinical queries feature supports evidence-based searching by allowing a specialized methodologic search for the highest levels of evidence in the literature on questions of therapy, diagnosis, etiology, prognosis, or clinical prediction guides (Fig. 5-4). This feature provides a quick check of the literature based on the Type of Question by

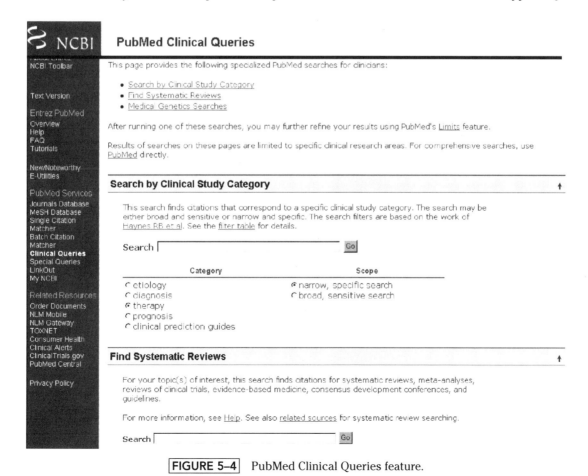

FIGURE 5–4   PubMed Clinical Queries feature.

using specialized filters to conduct a formulated search of key terms. Although it may not be as targeted as a PICO search, it allows for fast results on a topic. Clinical Queries also has a Systematic Review search, which allows one to search a topic of interest for secondary research. This feature looks for citations that include systematic reviews, meta-analysis, evidence-based reviews, and guidelines.

In addition to Clinical Queries, Special Queries allows one to limit the search for research in a specific subset. These include journals, topics, and interfaces. Examples of these are dental journals, AIDS or cancer, and TOXNET-toxicological databases.[8] These features are accessed by clicking on either Clinical Queries or Special Queries on the blue sidebar on the left-hand side of the screen.

Limits

The Limit feature (Fig. 5-5) allows for limiting the results of a search to specific fields, such as Age, Gender, Language, Type of Article (methodology), and subsets, such as Journal, Topics,

FIGURE 5–5 PubMed Limit feature.

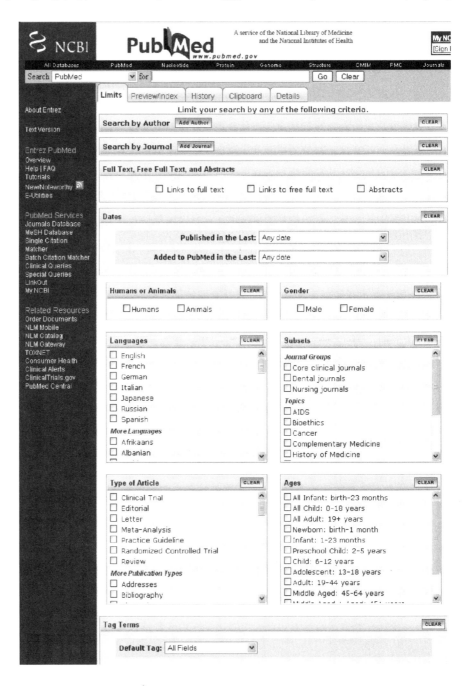

or Database. This feature is key to searching for levels of evidence because *Type of Article* allows the results to be limited to clinical trial, meta-analysis, practice guideline, randomized controlled trial, and review. However, there are some limitations of this feature when using the Review limitation. For example, the PubMed *Review* LIMIT feature includes all reviews, which does not allow a separation of specific types of reviews such as article, literature, academic, or systematic reviews. In addition, the meta-analysis LIMIT feature filters citations for quantitative summaries that combine results of independent studies, which also include systematic reviews. Thus systematic reviews can be indexed and found using either or both of these *Type of Article* LIMITs.

Boolean Operators

Boolean operators are words used to associate terms in a PubMed/MEDLINE search. They limit results of a search by allowing the combination of search terms or concepts. The three Boolean operators are **AND**, **OR**, and **NOT**, and must be capitalized when using them on PubMed.[9] The AND operator is used to retrieve results that contain all of the search terms in a citation (Fig. 5-6). A search for "Toothpaste AND Tooth bleaching" will retrieve only citations that reference both toothpaste and tooth bleaching. This should provide results of toothpaste that whiten or bleach teeth.

The OR operator looks for citations that have at least one of the terms and combines them together in one result. The OR operator is used to combine articles on similar topics or broaden the search (Fig. 5-7).

The NOT operator excludes the retrieval of terms from search results (Fig. 5-8). Typing "Toothpaste NOT Tooth bleaching" excludes results about bleaching, therefore focusing the results on only toothpastes without whitening effects. However, by using the NOT Boolean operator in this case, the results also may eliminate relevant citations that contain information about both toothpastes and bleaching.[9]

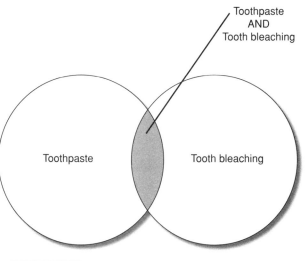

FIGURE 5–6 Boolean operator AND combines only sets that contain *both* terms.

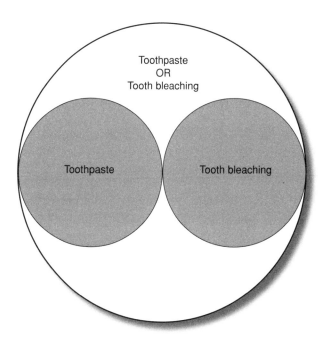

FIGURE 5–7 Boolean operator OR combines sets that contain at least one of the terms.

AN ANSWER FOR GAIL'S DRY MOUTH

Learning the skill to quickly access relevant research studies to answer a specific question takes time and patience. Proficiency comes through practice and experience. Using the PICO

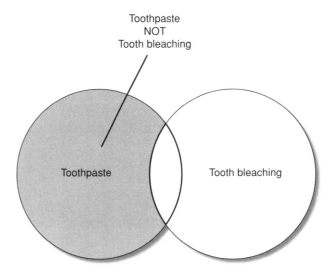

Toothpaste
NOT
Tooth bleaching

Toothpaste

Tooth bleaching

FIGURE 5–8 Boolean operator NOT excludes sets that contain the stated term even when it includes both terms.

question for Gail, this guidebook provides a step-by-step example that can be modeled when searching for answers to other PICO questions.

After having defined the PICO question, the strategy involved in conducting a PubMed search includes the following steps.

1. Identify the type of question (therapy/prevention, diagnosis, etiology/causation, or prognosis).
2. Identify the type of study/research methodology to search for (meta-analysis/systematic review, RCT, cohort study)
3. Identify alternate terms related to PICO question (synonyms for the problem, intervention, comparison, outcomes).
4. Identify MeSH terms for the PICO question (use the MeSH browser).
5. List the inclusion criteria limits.
6. Type the Intervention term(s) in the search box using the OR Boolean operator.
7. Combine it with the Patient/Problem/Population term using the appropriate Boolean operator (AND, OR, and/or NOT).
8. Limit the search by language and human subject (if applicable) (or age, gender, journal subsets).
9. Limit the search by publication type, beginning with the highest level of evidence (e.g., meta-analysis/ systematic review).
10. Review the citations and abstracts (the methodology often is included in the abstract).
11. Select citations that appear to address the question.
12. Access the related full-text articles or order them. (The full-text of articles for some journals are available via a link to the publisher's Web site from the PubMed abstract or citation display. If not, directions for ordering full-text copies of articles from a medical library [local fees and delivery methods may vary] or Loansome Doc are provided.[5])

To search for the evidence on PubMed, one may begin by using the Clinical Queries feature or the Find Systematic Reviews feature. In so doing, you may consider searching the topic "xerostomia" or xerostomia AND pilocarpine, the main intervention chosen for Gail.

The next step is to conduct an actual search on PubMed. The main topics and alternative terms identified on the *EBDM Worksheet* are used to identify MeSH terms. A completed EBDM Worksheet Part C is found in Fig. 5-9. By using the MeSH Browser on PubMed (accessed by clicking on MeSH Database located on the blue sidebar) the key MeSH terms that are related to the PICO question are identified and circled in Fig. 5-9. As stated earlier, using MeSH terms provides the most relevant results. If the MeSH terms do not provide sufficient results, then

EBDM Worksheet PART C

Completed Worksheet for Gail Case Example

Skill 2. Conducting a Computerized Search with Maximum Efficiency for Finding the Best External Evidence with which to Answer the Question

1. List main topics and alternate terms from your PICO question that can be used for your search. Circle MeSH Terms.

Dry mouth OR oral dryness	Salagen
(xerostomia)	bethanechol
salivary gland dysfunction	Urecholine
saliva stimulant	salivary flow
sialogogue	drug-induced
(pilocarpine)	

2. List your inclusion criteria: gender, age, year of publication, language / List irrelevant terms that you may want to exclude in your search

Human	Saliva substitute
English	
1966-present	

3. List where you plan to search (i.e., EBM Reviews, MEDLINE, PubMed, CINAHL, Cochrane).

MEDLINE/PubMed	
Cochrane Library	

4. List the Web addresses of the Internet search, and attach the information summary and web site evaluation. (See Chapter 7)

WEB SITE ADDRESS	INFORMATION FOUND
www.cochrane.org/reviews/index.htm (Cochrane collaboration)	Registered title: Nonpharmacological interventions for the management of xerostomia (title stage)

FIGURE 5–9 Completed EBDM Worksheet, Part C.

5. Include your search strategy. (Print from the PubMed History Tab.) or fill in the Table below

	Search History	Results
#1	Search pilocarpine OR bethanechol	8380
#2	Search drug-induced xerostomia	81
#3	Search #1 AND #2	3
#4	Search pilocarpine AND bethanechol	79
#5	Search #2 AND #4	0
#6	Search xerostomia	10464
#7	Search #4 AND #6	3
#8	Search #1 AND #6	233
#9	Search #1 AND #6 Limits: English, Humans	168
#10	Search #1 AND #6 Limits: English, Meta-Analysis, Humans	1
#11	Search #1 AND #6 Limits: English, Review, Humans	50
#12	Search #1 AND #6 Limits: English, Randomized Controlled Trial, Humans	33
#13	Search #1 AND #6 Limits: English, Clinical Trial, Humans	47
#14	Search #1 AND #6 Limits: English, Practice Guideline, Humans	0
#15		

FIGURE 5–9 Completed EBDM Worksheet, Part C, for Gail Case Example *(Continued)*

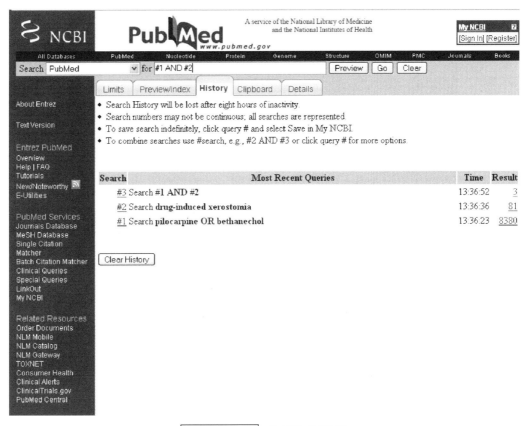

FIGURE 5-10 P AND (I OR C).

the words on the worksheet that do not have related MeSH terms can be searched as text words or the broader terms listed in the MeSH tree structure can be used.

After identifying the MeSH terms, begin the search by typing key words in the search box at the top of the PubMed homepage. The main key word for the Intervention is pilocarpine and the comparison is bethanechol as discussed previously. The patient's problem is drug-induced xerostomia. By connecting pilocarpine and the comparison bethanechol with the Boolean operator OR, the search retrieved 8,380 citations. By typing in drug-induced xerostomia, the search retrieves 81 citations. Combining these two searches with the Boolean operator AND retrieves 3 citations (Fig. 5-10). The citations include two relevant articles about both drug-induced xerostomia and pilocarpine for opioid-induced oral dryness in adults, which are very applicable to Gail's case (Fig. 5-11).

By combining the intervention with the comparison using the Boolean operator AND, the search should retrieve results that contain both therapies. Pilocarpine AND bethanechol retrieves 79 citations. However, by combining that with #2, drug-induced xerostomia, the results are zero. Searching for xerostomia alone retrieves 10,464 citations. By eliminating the descriptor "drug-induced," the search term xerostomia finds **more than 10,000 additional** citations related to relieving xerostomia. By combining the term xerostomia with #4 pilocarpine AND bethanechol, PubMed retrieves three citations that all seem relevant to Gail (Figs. 5-12 and 5-13).

Combining the intervention OR the comparison (Search #1) AND the P-main problem/patient description/population (Search #6), 233 citation are retrieved (Fig. 5-14). This number is too large to read through for relevance. By clicking on the Limits tab, one can access the PubMed Limit feature. It is best to use the Limits in stages by sorting the citations by language, human subjects, and then individual publication types to sort the citations by levels of evidence.

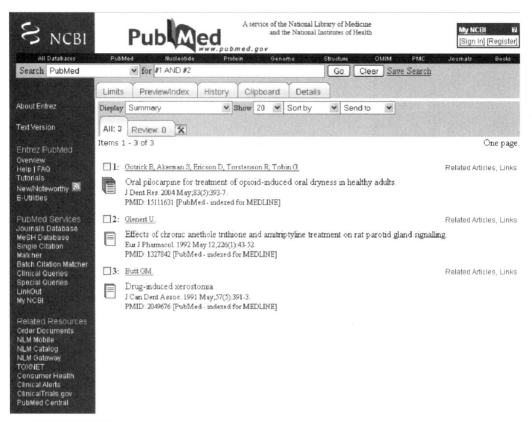

FIGURE 5–11 Results of drug-induced xerostomia AND (pilocarpine OR bethanechol).

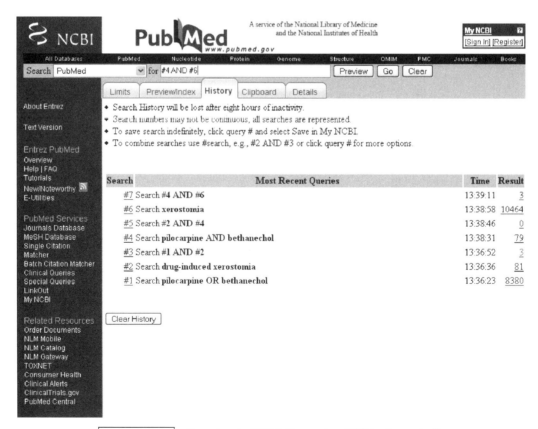

FIGURE 5–12 Xerostomia AND (pilocarpine AND bethanechol).

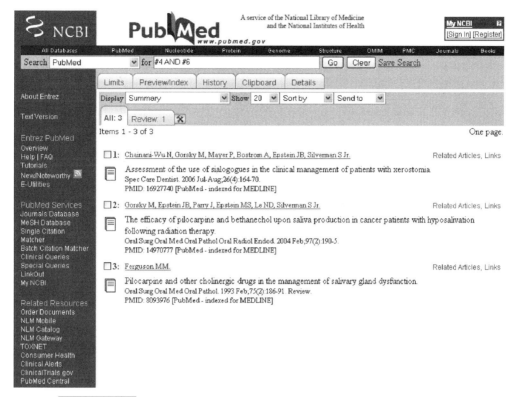

FIGURE 5–13   Results of xerostomia AND (pilocarpine AND bethanechol).

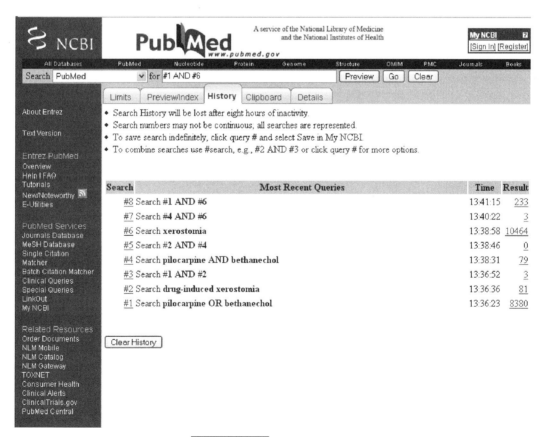

FIGURE 5–14   (I or C) AND P.

To limit search results, check the appropriate boxes that pertain to the search. First limit the results to Humans and English. This is done by checking English from the Languages menu, and Humans from the Humans or Animals menu (Fig. 5-15). Clicking on the word *GO* limits the search and displays the new results, thus reducing the number of citations from 233 to 168.

To now separate the results by levels of evidence, again click on the Limits feature. Remembering that there are two *Types of Articles* that will identify systematic reviews (meta-analysis and reviews), first select Meta-Analysis (Fig. 5-16) and click on *GO* to display the new results.

Of the remaining 138 citations, one meta-analysis is found: Treatment of xerostomia: a systematic review of therapeutic trials. *Dent Clin North Am*. 2002;46(4):847–856. Review. PMID: 12436835 (Fig. 5-17). Related links are listed to the right of the citation abstract. These provide hyperlinks to additional relevant articles that may answer Gail's question. So if only one great citation can be found, using this tool may pull up relevant evidence that may or may not have been provided in the search results.

Next, going back to the 168 citations and changing the publication types selection to Review, 50 citations are found. There are 33 RCTs, 47 clinical trials, and zero practice guidelines when those limits are applied. The search history is viewed by clicking on the History Tab in PubMed (Fig. 5-18).

In reviewing the citations and abstracts for these levels of evidence, we find that there are several citations that appear to answer the PICO question for Gail. Yet, to truly make an evidence-based decision regarding Gail, it is important to complete the EBDM process by retrieving the full text of the literature, critically appraising it, and determining if it applies to her specific question and situation before making the final decision. In this case, the first priority would be to read the systematic review of the therapeutic trials for the treatment of xerostomia. The second priority would be to look at the individual research/primary studies.

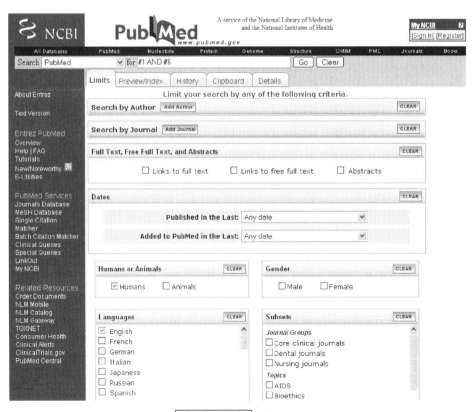

FIGURE 5–15 Limits.

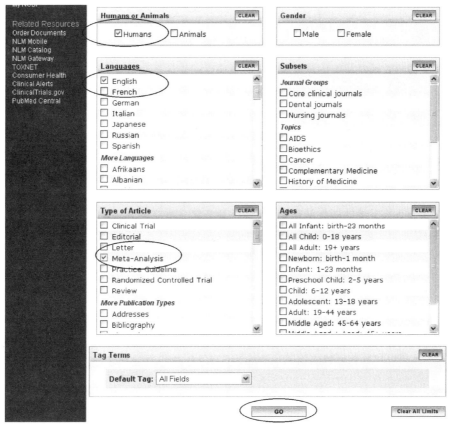

FIGURE 5–16 Limit to meta-analysis.

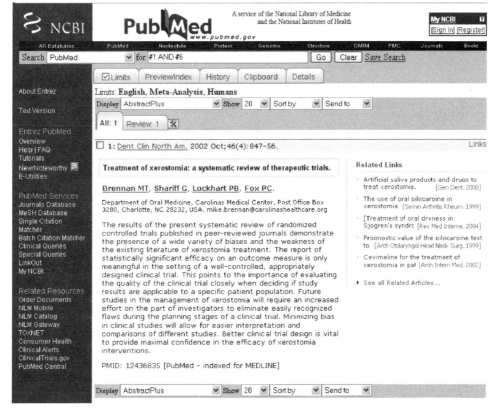

FIGURE 5–17 Results of meta-analysis limit.

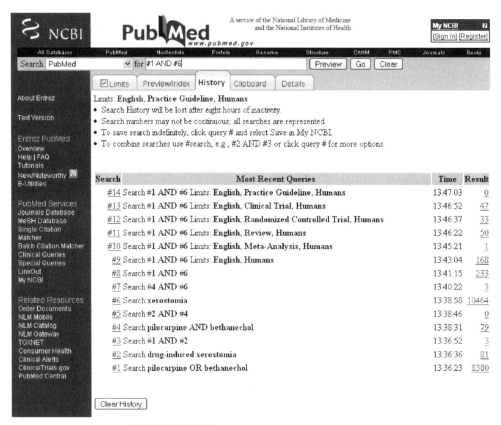

FIGURE 5–18   Final search history for Gail.

SEARCH STRATEGIES

Tables 5-2, 5-3, and 5-4 are examples of more comprehensive search strategies that combine the majority of search terms outlined in the EBDM worksheet for Gail. These are great practice. Try a search using these examples to fill in the results column.

TABLE 5–2

Combination of All Terms from the Worksheet (with the Exception of Drug-Induced)

	Search History	*Results*
#1	Xerostomia *OR* dry mouth *OR* oral dryness *OR* mouth dryness *OR* salivary gland dysfunction	
#2	Salagen *OR* pilocarpine *OR* bethanechol *OR* urecholine *OR* saliva stimulant *OR* salivary flow *OR* sialogogue	
#3	#1 and #2	
#4	Search #1 *AND* #2 Field: all fields, Limits: English, Human	
#5	Search #1 *AND* #2 Field: all fields, Limits: English, Meta-Analysis, Human	
#6	Search #1 *AND* #2 Field: all fields, Limits: English, Review, Human	
#7	Search #1 *AND* #2 Field: all fields, Limits: English, Randomized Controlled Trial, Human	
#8	Search #1 *AND* #2 Field: all fields, Limits: English, Clinical Trial, Human	
#9	Search #1 *AND* #2 Field: all fields, Limits: English, Practice Guideline, Human	

TABLE 5–3

Combination of the Patient Problem and Intervention for Gail

	Search History	Results
#1	Drug induced xerostomia *AND* pilocarpine	
#2	Xerostomia *AND* pilocarpine	
#2	Search #2 Field: all fields, Limits: English, Human	
#3	Search #2 Field: all fields, Limits: English, Meta-Analysis, Human	
	Related articles for PubMed (selected meta-analysis)	
#4	Search #2 Field: all fields, Limits: English, Review, Human	
#5	Search #2 Field: all fields, Limits: English, Randomized Controlled Trial, Human	
#6	Search #2 Field: all fields, Limits: English, Clinical Trial, Human	
#7	Search #2 Field: all fields, Limits: English, Practice Guideline, Human	

TABLE 5–4

Combination of the Patient Problem and Intervention *or* Comparison for Gail

	Search History	Results
#1	Xerostomia *OR* dry mouth *OR* oral dryness *OR* mouth dryness	
#2	Pilocarpine *OR* Salagen	
#3	Bethanechol *OR* urecholine	
#4	#2 *OR* #3	
#5	#1 *AND* #4	
#2	Search #2 Field: all fields, Limits: English, Human	
#3	Search #2 Field: all fields, Limits: English, Meta-Analysis, Human	
#4	Search #2 Field: all fields, Limits: English, Review, Human	
#5	Search #2 Field: all fields, Limits: English, Randomized Controlled Trial, Human	
#6	Search #2 Field: all fields, Limits: English, Clinical Trial, Human	
#7	Search #2 Field: all fields, Limits: English, Practice Guideline, Human	

Tables 5-5, 5-6, 5-7, and 5-8 provide templates for both simple and complex searches that may be helpful in shortening the learning curve for searching for relevant evidence on PubMed. These may be helpful when searching Pubmed for answers related to the cases in Exercise 5-1.

The outcomes are not included in this search because it was not necessary to use in order to limit the number of studies to a manageable size. The outcomes will be helpful during the critical appraisal step in determining if the study measures the objectives that are appropriate for the patient and their PICO question.

TABLE 5–5

Simplified Search History Template Problem and Intervention

	Search History Template
#1	P *AND* I
#2	Search #1 Field: all fields, Limits: English, Human
#3	Search #1 Field: all fields, Limits: English, Meta-Analysis, Human
#4	Search #1 Field: all fields, Limits: English, Review, Human
#5	Search #1 Field: all fields, Limits: English, Randomized Controlled Trial, Human
#6	Search #1 Field: all fields, Limits: English, Clinical Trial, Human
#7	Search #1 Field: all fields, Limits: English, Practice Guideline, Human

TABLE 5–6

Complex Search History Template Problem and Intervention

	Search History Template
#1	P *OR* term *OR* term *OR* term *OR* term
#2	I *OR* term *OR* term *OR* term *OR* term *OR* term
#3	#1 *AND* #2
#4	Search #3 Field: all fields, Limits: English, Human
#5	Search #3 Field: all fields, Limits: English, Meta-Analysis, Human
#6	Search #3 Field: all fields, Limits: English, Review, Human
#7	Search #3 Field: all fields, Limits: English, Randomized Controlled Trial, Human
#8	Search #3 Field: all fields, Limits: English, Clinical Trial, Human
#9	Search #3 Field: all fields, Limits: English, Practice Guideline, Human

TABLE 5–7

Simplified Search History Template Problem, Intervention, Comparison

	Search History Template
#1	I *OR* C
#2	P
#3	#1 *AND* #2
#4	Search #3 Field: all fields, Limits: English, Human
#5	Search #3 Field: all fields, Limits: English, Meta-Analysis, Human
#6	Search #3 Field: all fields, Limits: English, Review, Human
#7	Search #3 Field: all fields, Limits: English, Randomized Controlled Trial, Human
#8	Search #3 Field: all fields, Limits: English, Clinical Trial, Human
#9	Search #3 Field: all fields, Limits: English, Practice Guideline, Human

TABLE 5-8

Complex Search History Template Problem, Intervention, Comparison

	Search History Template
#1	P *OR* term *OR* term *OR* term *OR* term
#2	I *OR* term *OR* term *OR* term *OR* term *OR* term
#3	C *OR* term *OR* term *OR* term *OR* term *OR* term
#4	#2 *OR* #3
#5	#1 *AND* #4
#6	Search #5 Field: all fields, Limits: English, Human
#7	Search #5 Field: all fields, Limits: English, Meta-Analysis, Human
#8	Search #5 Field: all fields, Limits: English, Review, Human
#9	Search #5 Field: all fields, Limits: English, Randomized Controlled Trial, Human
#10	Search #5 Field: all fields, Limits: English, Clinical Trial, Human
#11	Search #5 Field: all Fields, Limits: English, Practice Guideline, Human

CONCLUSION

Key tips to keep in mind:

- Keep the search simple
- Try to limit the search terms to the key terms identified in the PICO question
- The MeSH browser often helps clarify terms and identify better word choices
- The Limit feature allows quick elimination based on language, subject; and level of evidence

Searching for evidence requires new information retrieval skills in order to take full advantage of the capabilities that PubMed and other databases provide. Learning how these are structured, their language, and searching rules increases your abilities and success in finding relevant evidence. As with learning any new skills, searching for valid evidence using online databases can be frustrating. However, with a little time and practice, they can be mastered so that the best evidence can be accessed with maximum efficiency.

The EBDM Worksheet provides a framework for learning the needed skills related to each aspect of the evidence-based decision-making process. Filling out the EBDM Worksheet guides you through structuring the PICO question and identifying search terms, the type of study methodology related to the question, and inclusion criteria and provides an outline used to search the literature that will provide relevant evidence to answer the PICO question. Keep in mind there is not a perfect format for conducting an effective search. There is more than one way to find evidence to answer a question, depending on the number and specificity of terms used and the sequence in limiting results and combining terms using Boolean operators. The procedures outlined here provide an introduction to learning how to conduct an efficient search and a basic example of how to apply the key features of PubMed to obtain evidence to answer Gail's question and the patient cases that were introduced in Chapter 2.

REFERENCES

1. Cochrane Collaboration. What is the Cochrane Collaboration. Cochrane Collaboration Web site. www.cochrane.org. Accessed July 19, 2006.
2. Cochrane Collection. Cochrane Collaboration—Cochrane entities. Cochrane Collaboration Web site. www.cochrane.org. Accessed July 19, 2006.
3. Ovid scope note for CINAHL. Ovid Technologies Web site. www.usc.edu/ovid. Accessed July 19, 2006.
4. CINAHL. Products and services. CINAHL Database Web site. www.cinahl.com/prodsvcs/prodsvcs.htm. Accessed July 19, 2006.
5. National Library of Medicine, NCBI. PubMed. National Library of Medicine, NIH, 2001. PubMed overview Web site. www.ncbi.nlm.nih.gov/entrez/query/static/overview.html. Accessed July 19, 2006.
6. Ovid scope note for PubMed. Ovid Technologies Web site. www.usc.edu/ovid. Accessed July 19, 2006.
7. National Library of Medicine, NCBI. PubMed. National Library of Medicine, NIH, 2001. PubMed MeSH browser Web site. www.nlm.nih.gov/mesh/MBrowser.html. Accessed July 19, 2006.
8. National Library of Medicine, NCBI. PubMed. National Library of Medicine, NIH, 2001. PubMed clinical queries Web site. www.ncbi.nlm.nih.gov/entrez/query/static/clinical.shtml. Accessed July 19, 2006.
9. National Library of Medicine. PubMed Tutorial. PubMed online training. National Library of Medicine, NIH, 2001. PubMed tutorial Web site. www.nlm.nih.gov/bsd/disted/pubmed.html. Accessed July 19, 2006.

SUGGESTED ACTIVITIES

At this time, complete the quiz. Then answer the critical thinking questions. Next, complete Exercise 5-1 to strengthen the second skill of the EBDM process: Conducting a computerized search with maximum efficiency for finding the best external evidence with which to answer the question.

QUIZ

1. When using PubMed, the proper Boolean operator to exclude terms from your search is:
   a. not
   b. NOT
   c. or
   d. OR
2. To filter the citations according to type of study, use this feature of PubMed:
   a. History
   b. Subsets
   c. Publication dates
   d. Limits
3. To access the search history page, that lists your search strategy, you must click here (please circle where to click to access the search strategy).

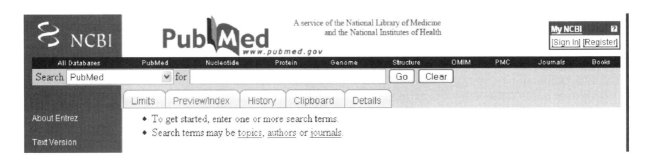

4. To filter the citations to randomized controlled trials, circle where you would click.

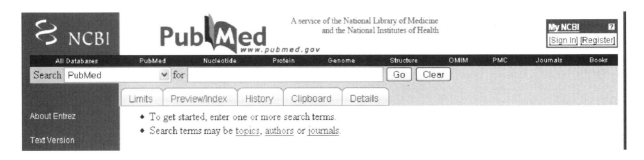

5. Match the terms with the most appropriate database in which to search.

_____ MeSH	A. Cochrane Database
_____ American Nurses Association	B. PubMed/Medline
_____ Systematic review	C. CINAHL

CRITICAL THINKING QUESTIONS

1. Why are MeSH terms helpful when searching MEDLINE?

2. Describe one new aspect of PubMed learned after completing the PubMed tutorial. How will this help you answer clinical questions more effectively?

3. Compare and contrast two of the biomedical databases introduced in this section.

EXERCISE 5-1

Fill out Part C of the EBDM Worksheet for each of the 5 cases which will guide the searching process to find the best evidence to answer the PICO questions for Morty, Trevor, Dr. Bailer, Jennifer, and Sam. Define your search terms for each case and identify inclusion criteria (Limits) and where you plan to search. Then search the literature to find evidence to answer the question for each case. Start with a simplified search using just the Problem and Intervention. Then add the comparison to further limit the search. If the results are too small, then increase the search field by combining the alternate terms with the PICO terms. Search History Templates are provided in Tables 5-5 to 5-8 and can be used as a guide to getting started. When using the limits, click on the Limits tab and check the appropriate boxes to limit each field rather than typing the limits as seen in the search history examples. Print your search history from PubMed.

Morty

Mr. Morty Kramer, a 55-year-old man, has been using unwaxed floss his whole life and flosses frequently. At his last dental appointment, he was treated by a new hygienist, who told him that he needed to change to using a waxed floss because it is more effective in removing plaque. Morty is happy with his current oral hygiene regimen and asks if he really needs to change.

Trevor

Trevor is a 27-year-old bartender who has used chewing tobacco for 13 years. He is a frequent user who chews almost 5 hours a day. He has just learned from his oral health care provider that he has developed precancerous lesions in the vestibular area where he holds the tobacco plug. This new information has motivated him to quit. Trevor knows he can't quit by willpower alone because he has tried in the past. He wants to know if a non-nicotine aid in tobacco cessation is helpful in this endeavor, or if a nicotine patch is better in helping users permanently quit. He would like to know if behavioral therapy/counseling might help.

Dr. Bailer

Dr. Bailer recently graduated from dental school and is building a new dental practice. As he designs his building, he is trying to decide whether to purchase digital radiograph equipment or to use traditional radiography. He is interested in knowing the most accurate method for caries detection.

Jennifer

Your morning patient, Mrs. Jennifer Morris, comes to you distressed because of an article she read on the Internet about the dangers of mercury in her amalgam restorations. She is worried that her seven amalgam fillings are poisoning her. She is very concerned not only for her own health, but for her two young daughters who also have amalgam restorations. Jennifer doesn't want to replace her fillings if it isn't necessary, but needs proof that she and her children are going to be healthy.

To reassure your patient, you give her advice based on your clinical experience and judgment; however, she still seems very upset and troubled. You inform her that you will do a thorough search of the current scientific literature and get back to her with your findings. She seems more relaxed with this thought and leaves eager to hear from you soon.

Sam

Sam is a 49-year-old man with moderate periodontitis, who was recently diagnosed with type 2 diabetes mellitus. Sam's glycosylated hemoglobin (HbA1) is 12%, which places him in the category of poorly controlled diabetes. Sam is worried that his diabetes will increase his chance of losing his teeth. He wants to know the effect and impact diabetes now has on his oral health.

Name_____Topic_____

EBDM Worksheet Part C

*Skill 2. Conducting a Computerized Search with Maximum Efficiency for Finding the Best
External Evidence with which to Answer the Question*

1. List main topics and alternate terms from your PICO question that can be used for your search.
   Circle MeSH Terms.

   _____   _____
   _____   _____
   _____   _____
   _____   _____
   _____   _____
   _____   _____

2. List your inclusion criteria: gender,   List irrelevant terms that you may
   age, year of publication, language   want to exclude in your search

   _____   _____
   _____   _____
   _____   _____
   _____   _____
   _____   _____

3. List where you plan to search (i.e., EBM Reviews, MEDLINE, PubMed, CINAHL, Cochrane)

   _____   _____
   _____   _____
   _____   _____

4. List the Web addresses of the Internet search and attach the information summary and Web site
   evaluation. (See Chapter 7.)

   WEB SITE ADDRESS   INFORMATION FOUND
   _____   _____
   _____   _____
   _____   _____
   _____   _____
   _____   _____
   _____   _____
   _____   _____
   _____   _____

Name_____Topic_____

EBDM Worksheet Part C (continued)

5. Include your search strategy. Print from the PubMed "History" tab or fill in the table.

	Search History	Results
#1		
#2		
#3		
#4		
#5		
#6		
#7		
#8		
#9		
#10		
#11		
#12		
#13		
#14		
#15		

CHAPTER 6

Critical Appraisal of the Evidence

Critically Appraising the Evidence for its Validity and Usefulness (Clinical Applicability).

PURPOSE

The purpose of this section is to discuss critical appraisal criteria and the evaluation tools that simplify the process of determining the credibility and usefulness of the evidence. These tools can be used to assess the methodologic quality of a study and assist in making initial judgments. A case scenario will demonstrate how to determine the validity of the study by examining the strengths and weaknesses of how the study was conducted.

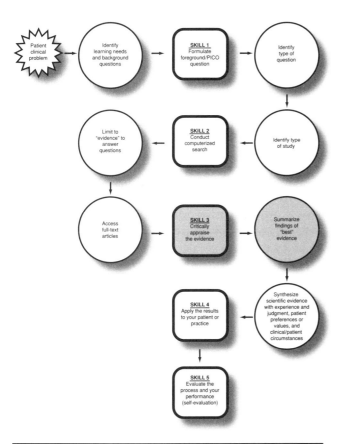

OBJECTIVES

After completing this chapter, readers will be able to:

1. Identify key questions in the critical appraisal process

2. Critique different study methodologies, such as randomized controlled trials and systematic reviews, using international guidelines and evaluation tools:
   - CASP (Critical Appraisal Skills Programme)
   - CONSORT (Consolidated Standards of Reporting Trials—RCTs)
   - QUOROM (Quality Of Reporting Of Meta-analyses)
   - STARD (Standards for Reporting of Diagnostic Accuracy)
   - MOOSE (Meta-analysis of Observational Studies in Epidemiology)

SUGGESTED ACTIVITIES

Quiz
Critical Thinking Questions
Exercise 6-1

KEY QUESTIONS IN APPRAISING THE SCIENTIFIC LITERATURE

Having an understanding of research design provides the foundation necessary for the critical appraisal process. However, for many practitioners, the skills for evaluating research studies are not second nature. Fortunately, evidence-based groups have developed international guidelines and the tools to assist in critical appraisal of the evidence.[1-4] These tools consist of a structured series of questions or items that help review the validity of the study. **Validity** is defined by the *Users' Guides to the Medical Literature* as the degree to which a study appropriately answers the question being asked or an instrument measures what it is suppose to measure and performs the functions that it purports to perform. Validity is often referenced as it relates to **bias**—systematic deviations from the underlying truth.[1]

Do not confuse validity with reliability. Reliability refers to the consistency of a set of measurements or a measuring instrument. That is, a test instrument is said to be reliable if it yields consistent results over repeated tests of the same subject under ideal conditions. However, just because a test or instrument is reliable does not mean it is valid. For example, if an explorer is used to measure pocket depth, the same results may be obtained over and over. However, an explorer is not a valid instrument to measure pocket depth. When evaluating test instruments, validity is more important than reliability; however, to be useful, there must be both reasonable validity and reliability.

For the most part, the Journal of the American Medical Association (JAMA) Series of articles on the *Users' Guides to the Medical Literature*, prepared by the Evidence-Based Medicine Working Group,[1] serve as the basis for these checklists. One group, CASP (the Critical Appraisal Skills Programme) offers online downloadable learning resources including Web-based and PDF checklists to appraise systematic reviews (SRs), randomized controlled trial (RCTs), cohort studies, case control studies, and diagnostic test studies. The CASP checklists consist of a structured series of YES/NO questions that are based on three key questions:[2,3,5]

1. Are the results of the study valid?
2. What are the results?
3. Will the results help in caring for my patient?

A subset of more detailed questions exists for each of the three key questions, which further helps determine the validity, results, and applicability of the evidence.[2] In addition to the subset of questions, most of the checklists include helpful hints as to what the questions mean. For example, under *Are the results of the study valid?* and the subset question *Did the trial address a clearly focused research question?*, a helpful hint is provided on what "focused" can mean (i.e., in terms of the population studied, the intervention given, and the outcomes considered). Table 6-1 illustrates the three key questions and the related subset of questions for each type of question: therapy/prevention, harm/etiology/causation, prognosis, and diagnosis. This table is followed by Table 6-2, which illustrates how a CASP form would be completed for an RCT related to the Gail case.

The key questions are important in that they assist practitioners in determining if they can place confidence in the results. For example, in reviewing *Are the results of the study valid?*, it is important to know the specific question addressed and if it was reasonable. How patients are recruited, randomly assigned, and treated throughout the study indicates if the methods used minimize bias and are reproducible.

The characteristics of an individual RCT parallel the information that should be known about a systematic review in terms of knowing the criteria for including or excluding studies from the review. In looking at whether the review included the right type of studies, it is important to review the quality of those studies since differences in study methods could explain important differences among results and the interpretation of the intervention's benefit.[8,9] Having consistent results from studies whose methods were weak (observational studies vs. RCTs) should raise questions because they tend to overestimate the effectiveness of treatment and prevention interventions,[9] as was demonstrated in observational studies on the use of hormonal replacement therapy.[10] In this case, observational studies found lower rates of coronary heart disease (CHD) in women who take postmenopausal estrogen than in women who do not. However, this benefit was not confirmed in clinical trials, which are more rigorously designed and controlled, minimize bias, and provide a higher level of evidence.

Subsequently, the Heart and Estrogen/Progestin Replacement Study (HERS) was conducted to determine if estrogen plus progestin therapy alters the risk for CHD events in postmenopausal women with established coronary disease. The outcome of this study was that the treatment did not reduce the overall rate of CHD events in postmenopausal women with established coronary disease, whereas the treatment did increase the rate of thromboembolic events and gallbladder disease. Based on the finding of no overall cardiovascular benefit and a pattern of early increase in risk of CHD events, treatment was not recommended for the purpose of secondary prevention of CHD.[10]

In an effort to improve the quality of published research, several international guidelines have been published for the reporting of research studies. These include the **CONSORT** statement (Consolidated Standards of Reporting Trials),[4] which is designed to improve the quality of reporting randomized clinical trials, and **QUOROM** (the Quality of Reporting of Meta-analyses), designed to improve the reporting of SRs.[11] These guidelines and flow charts help guarantee the integrity of the reported results and also serve as criteria that clinicians can use for evaluating an RCT or SR. The CONSORT guidelines are presented in Table 6-3 and the QUOROM guidelines are presented in Table 6-4. The online version of the CONSORT checklist links to an explanation of each criterion should the user need further information. Unlike the CASP forms that use a YES/NO format, the CONSORT and QUOROM forms ask the reviewer to list the page number where the information was reported.

The CONSORT statement is available in several languages and has been endorsed by prominent medical journals such as *The Lancet, Annals of Internal Medicine*, and the *Journal of the American Medical Association* and most recently, the *New England Journal of Medicine*. The *New England Journal of Medicine* now requests authors to provide a flow diagram in CONSORT format and all of the information required by the CONSORT checklist when reporting on clinical trials.[12] These requirements assist in standardizing the peer-review process as well as help practitioners understand the experimental process so that they can evaluate the validity of the

TABLE 6-1

Critical Analysis Questions[2,5,6]

Type of Question	Therapy/Prevention	Rationale	Diagnosis	Prognosis	Harm/Etiology/Causation
Type of study	RCT, cohort study, SR/MA of RCTs, SR/MA of cohort studies		Prospective cohort study MA or SR of controlled trials, single controlled trial	Meta-analysis or SR of inception cohort studies, cohort study	Meta-analysis or SR of RCTs, single RCT SR of cohort studies Single cohort study
Key questions: Are the results of the study (trial) valid?	Did the trial or *review* address a clearly focused question?	If the trial is too broad it may not provide an accurate picture of the therapy.	Were the right patients enrolled in the study that was representative of those with the clinical problem?	Was there a defined, representative sample of patients assembled at a common (usually early) point in the course of their disease and free of the outcome of interest?	Were there clearly defined groups of patients, similar in all important ways other than exposure to the treatment or other cause?
Is it worth continuing?	Is a trial (RCT) an appropriate method to answer this issue? *Did the review include the appropriate type of studies?*	As discussed in Section 4, the study design should match the methodology.	Was there a clearly identified comparison group, at least one of which was free from the target disorder?	Were the patients sufficiently similar in regard to prognostic risk?	Were treatments/exposures and clinical outcomes measured in the same ways in the groups being compared (was the assessment of outcomes either objective or blinded to exposure)?
	How were patients assigned to treatment groups? *Did reviewers identify all relevant studies?*	This method should be rigorous to eliminate potential bias.	Was there an independent, blind comparison with a reference ("gold") standard of diagnosis?	Was there follow-up of at least 80% of the patient until the occurrence of either a major study endpoint or end of the study?	Was the follow-up of study patients sufficiently complete?

(Continued)

TABLE 6–1

(Continued)

Type of question	Therapy/Prevention	Diagnosis	Prognosis	Harm/Etiology/Causation
Were participants, staff, and study personnel "blinded" to groups and treatment? *Did reviewers assess the quality of included studies?*	Again, the data collection and treatment allocation should reflect rigorous methods to maintain quality and minimize bias.	Was the reference standard applied regardless of the diagnostic test result? Was the diagnostic process credible?	Were objective and unbiased outcome criteria applied in a "blinded" fashion?	Do the results satisfy some "diagnostic tests for causation"? • Is it clear that the exposure preceded the onset of the outcome? • Is there a dose-response gradient? • Is there positive evidence from a "dechallenge-rechallenge" study? • Is the association consistent from study to study?
Were all the participants who entered the trial properly accounted for at its conclusion? *If the results of the studies were combined, was it reasonable to do so?*	Participants that do not complete the study can skew the results and for the SR- data should compare apples to apples and oranges to oranges.	For initially undiagnosed patients, was follow-up sufficiently long and complete?	If subgroups with different prognoses are identified, was there adjustment for important prognostic factors?	Does the association make biologic sense?
Aside from the experimental intervention, were the groups treated in the same way?	The elimination of additional variables provides a more accurate result.	Was the test (or cluster of tests) validated in a second, independent group of patients?	Was there validation in an independent group ("test set") of patients?	Did both groups retain a similar prognosis after the start of the study?
Did the study have enough participants to minimize the play of chance?	Sample size is important. Validity is increased with larger sample sizes.			

(Continued)

TABLE 6–1
(Continued)

Type of question	Therapy/Prevention		Diagnosis	Prognosis	Harm/Etiology/Causation
What are the results? **Is it worth continuing?**	How are the results presented? What is the main result?	The results should be presented in appropriate measurements and values for the methods the study was conducted.	What were the diagnoses and their probabilities?	Over time, how likely are the outcomes?	How strong is the association between outcome and exposure?
	How precise are these results? (*p* values and confidence intervals)	The values should show statistical significance. Are the values also clinically relevant?	How precise are the estimates of disease probability?	How precise are the estimates of likelihood?	How precise is the estimate of risk?
Will the results help in caring for my patient?	Can the results be applied to my patient?	The likelihood of attaining the same results may increase when the study population closely resembles your patient	These questions will be covered in depth in Chapter 8.	These questions will be covered in depth in Chapter 8.	These questions will be covered in depth in Chapter 8.
	Were all important outcomes considered?	It is valuable to look at outcomes that reflect the patients' culture, values, and beliefs.			

Adapted from CASP Appraisal Tools: www.phru.nhs.uk/casp/critical_appraisal_tools.htm and the Users' Guides to the Medical Literature, www.cche.net/usersguides/therapy.asp and www.cche.net/usersguides/overview.asp

---

TABLE 6–2

CASP Critical Appraisal of an RCT for Gail: Oral Pilocarpine for Treatment of Opioid-Induced Oral Dryness in Healthy Adults, by Gotrick B et al.[7]

Critical Appraisal Skills Programme (CASP)
Making sense of evidence
10 questions to help you make sense of randomized controlled trials

....

Screening questions

1. Did the study ask a clearly focused question? ☐ Yes ☑ Can't tell ☐ No ☐
   Consider if the question is "focused" in terms of:
   – *the population studied*
   – *the intervention given*
   – *the outcomes considered*

....

2. Was this a randomised controlled trial (RCT) ☐ Yes ☑ Can't tell ☐ No ☐
   and was it appropriately so?
   Consider:
   – *why this study was carried out as an RCT*
   – *if this was the right research approach for the question being asked*
   Is it worth continuing?

....

Detailed questions

....

3. Were participants appropriately allocated to ☐ Yes ☑ Can't tell ☐ No ☐
   intervention and control groups?
   Consider:
   – *how participants were allocated to intervention and control groups. Was the process truly random?*
   – *whether the method of allocation was described. Was a method used to balance the randomization (e.g., stratification)?*
   – *how the randomization schedule was generated and how a participant was allocated to a study group*
   – *if the groups were well balanced. Are any differences between the groups at entry to the trial reported?*
   – *if there were differences reported that might have explained any outcome(s) (confounding)*

....

4. Were participants, staff and study personnel ☐ Yes ☑ Can't ☐ tell No ☐
   "blind" to participants' study group?
   Consider:
   – *the fact that blinding is not always possible*
   – *if every effort was made to achieve blinding*
   – *if you think it matters in this study*
   – *the fact that we are looking for "observer bias"*

....

5. Were all of the participants who entered the ☐ Yes ☑ Can't tell ☐ No ☐
   trial accounted for at its conclusion?
   Consider:
   – *if any intervention-group participants got a control-group option or vice versa*
   – *if all participants were followed up in each study group (was there loss-to-follow-up?)*
   – *if all the participants' outcomes were analyzed by the groups to which they were originally allocated (intention-to-treat analysis)*
   – *what additional information would you like to have seen to make you feel better about this*

....

(Continued)

TABLE 6-2

(Continued)

6. Were the participants in all groups followed ☐ Yes ☑ Can't tell ☐ No ☐ up and data collected in the same way?
   Consider:
   –if, for example, they were reviewed at the same time intervals and if they received the same amount of attention from researchers and health workers. Any differences may introduce performance bias.

....

7. Did the study have enough participants to ☐ Yes ☑ Can't tell ☐ No ☐ minimize the play of chance?
   Consider:
   – if there is a power calculation. This will estimate how many participants are needed to be reasonably sure of finding something important (if it really exists and for a given level of uncertainty about the final result)

....

8. How are the results presented and what is the main result?
   Consider:
   – if, for example, the results are presented as a proportion of people experiencing an outcome, such as risks, or as a measurement, such as mean or median differences, or as survival curves and hazards
   – how large this size of result is and how meaningful it is
   – how you would sum up the bottom-line result of the trial in one sentence

Actual flow rates of unstimulated whole saliva
Subjective "sensation" of flow of saliva

....

9. How precise are these results?
   Consider:
   – if the result is precise enough to make a decision
   – if a confidence interval were reported. Would your decision about whether or not to use this intervention be the same at the upper confidence limit as at the lower confidence limit?
   – if a p value is reported where confidence intervals are unavailable

   p value reported and confidence interval is 95%

....

10. Were all important outcomes considered so ☐ Yes ☑ Can't tell ☐ No ☐ the results can be applied?
    Consider whether:
    – the people included in the trial could be different from your population in ways that would produce different results
    – your local setting differs much from that of the trial
    – you can provide the same treatment in your setting

    Consider outcomes from the point of view of the:
    – individual
    – policy maker and professionals
    – family/caregivers
    – wider community

    Consider whether:
    – any benefit reported outweighs any harm and/or cost. If this information is not reported can it be filled in from elsewhere?
    – policy or practice should change as a result of the evidence contained in this trial

....

TABLE 6-3

CONSORT Checklist of Items to Include When Reporting a Randomized Trial[4]

Paper Section and Topic	Item	Description	Reported on Page No.
Title and abstract	1	How participants were allocated to interventions (e.g., "random allocation," "randomized," "randomly assigned").	
Introduction Background	2	Scientific background and explanation of rationale.	
Methods Participants	3	Eligibility criteria for participants and the settings and locations where the data were collected.	
Interventions	4	Precise details of the interventions intended for each group and how and when they were actually administered.	
Objectives	5	Specific objectives and hypotheses.	
Outcomes	6	Clearly defined primary and secondary outcome measures and, when applicable, any methods used to enhance the quality of measurements (e.g., multiple observations, training of assessors).	
Sample size	7	How sample size was determined and, when applicable, explanation of any interim analyses and stopping rules.	
Randomization— sequence generation	8	Method used to generate the random allocation sequence, including details of any restrictions (e.g., blocking, stratification)	
Randomization— allocation concealment	9	Method used to implement the random allocation sequence (e.g., numbered containers, central telephone), clarifying whether the sequence was concealed until interventions were assigned.	
Randomization— implementation	10	Who generated the allocation sequence, who enrolled participants, and who assigned participants to their groups.	
Blinding (masking)	11	Whether or not participants, those administering the interventions, and those assessing the outcomes were blinded to group assignment. When relevant, how the success of blinding was evaluated.	
Statistical methods	12	Statistical methods used to compare groups for primary outcome(s); methods for additional analyses, such as subgroup analyses and adjusted analyses.	
Results Participant flow	13	Flow of participants through each stage (a diagram is strongly recommended). Specifically, for each group report the numbers of participants randomly assigned, receiving intended treatment, completing the study protocol, and analyzed for the primary outcome. Describe protocol deviations from study as planned, together with reasons.	
Recruitment	14	Dates defining the periods of recruitment and follow-up.	
Baseline data	15	Baseline demographic and clinical characteristics of each group.	
Numbers analyzed	16	Number of participants (denominator) in each group included in each analysis and whether the analysis was by "intention-to-treat." State the results in absolute numbers when feasible (e.g., 10/20, not 50%).	
Outcomes and estimation	17	For each primary and secondary outcome, a summary of results for each group, and the estimated effect size and its precision (e.g., 95% confidence interval).	

(Continued)

TABLE 6–3

(Continued)

Paper Section and Topic	Item	Description	Reported on Page No.
Ancillary analyses	18	Address multiplicity by reporting any other analyses performed, including subgroup analyses and adjusted analyses, indicating those prespecified and those exploratory.	
Adverse events	19	All important adverse events or side effects in each intervention group.	
Discussion Interpretation	20	Interpretation of the results, taking into account study hypotheses, sources of potential bias or imprecision and the dangers associated with multiplicity of analyses, and outcomes.	
Generalizability	21	Generalizability (external validity) of the trial findings.	
Overall evidence	22	General interpretation of the results in the context of current evidence.	

http://www.consort–statement.org

TABLE 6–4

QUOROM Guidelines for Reporting Systematic Reviews[11]

Section	Content Description
Structured abstract	• Objectives—specific clinical question • Data sources • Review methods • Results—randomized controlled trial characteristics and data analysis • Conclusions—main results
Introduction	• Explicit clinical problem, intervention, and rationale
Methods	• Searching—information sources • Selection—inclusion and exclusion criteria for selecting studies • Validity assessment—criteria and process used • Data abstraction—processes used • Study characteristics—design type, intervention, and outcome details • Quantitative data synthesis—measures of effect, statistical assessment
Results	• Trial flow • Study characteristics—presentation of data for each RCT • Quantitative data synthesis—report on the selection and validity, summary results
Discussion	• Summary of key findings, discussion of clinical validity • Interpretation of results based on totality of available evidence • Description of potential biases • Future research agenda suggestions

http://www.consort–statement.org

study and interpret the clinical importance of the overall results.

Another facet of reporting should include the source of funding. For example, this could be grant funding from federal agencies, professional associations, or contracts from private industry. Again, researchers will want to thoroughly report each aspect of their study to demonstrate how bias is minimized or eliminated.

In addition to the criteria for reporting RCTs and SRs, criteria for improving the reporting of diagnostic studies, **STARD** (the Standards for Reporting of Diagnostic Accuracy)[13] were developed as were **MOOSE** (Meta-analysis of Observational Studies in Epidemiology)[14] for improving the reporting of studies of etiology or effectiveness (Appendices 6-A and 6-B). MOOSE criteria cover studies that use data from an existing database as well as those that use a cross-sectional, a case series, a case control, historical controls, or a cohort design. Again, the purpose of the criteria is to help readers judge the potential for bias in the study and to appraise the applicability of the findings.

APPRAISING THE EVIDENCE FOR GAIL: A SYSTEMATIC REVIEW

In Chapter 2, Asking Good Questions, the PICO question for Gail was defined as:

> In a patient with xerostomia, will pilocarpine as compared to bethanechol increase salivary flow and decrease dry mouth?

To answer the question, begin with the highest level of evidence that can be found. In this case, it is the SR by Brennan et al. titled, "Treatment of xerostomia: a systematic review of therapeutic trials."[15] Even though a SR or meta-analysis represents already appraised and synthesized studies that investigate the same question, it is necessary to review the evidence to determine if the methods were conducted rigorously and appropriately. Also, remember the strength of the evidence derived from the SR depends on the quality of the previously published original studies. The QUOROM form was used to evaluate the credibility of the SR. A completed QUOROM evaluation of this SR is found in Table 6-5.

Discussion of the SR Critical Appraisal for Gail

The main flaw of this SR is that the purpose was to simply rate the level of evidence of the available RCTs for the management of xerostomia rather than to determine the best treatment for xerostomia. Results showed four "Level A" evidence RCTs that studied pilocarpine as the treatment for xerostomia. These studies are summarized; however, it may have been more beneficial if the authors had spent more time in synthesizing the results of these four studies and the five "Level B" studies to form a conclusion about the "best evidence" treatment of xerostomia. However, that was not the stated purpose of the SR.

APPRAISING THE EVIDENCE FOR GAIL: RCTs

The CASP form in Table 6-2 reviewed the RCT, *Oral pilocarpine for treatment of opioid-induced oral dryness in healthy adults*.[7] The CONSORT form is used to evaluate *The efficacy of pilocarpine and bethanechol upon saliva production in cancer patients with hyposalivation following radiation therapy*, by Gorsky et al.,[16] because of its acceptance as an international guideline and its relative ease to use, even for someone without a research methodology background. This analysis is summarized in Table 6-6. After the review of the evidence for Gail's question is completed, the findings are ready to be discussed with her. This will be presented in Chapter 8.

Discussion of the RCT Critical Appraisal for Gail

The background and purpose of the study were written clearly; however, details in the methods section are lacking. For example, it is not clear where the study took place, how patients were recruited, and how patients were assigned to study groups. Also, a chart diagramming the flow of patients was not available that would have clarified the number of groups and who received only one treatment and who participated in the crossover arm of the study. Baseline and follow-up measurements were clearly defined, as were the results and discussion. Based on this analysis of the study, the reader must either assume that appropriate procedures were followed and therefore accept the results or question the results and whether they are reasonable given the information that is presented. Although the study is well written in terms of readability, the CONSORT guidelines demonstrate how the reporting of the study could be strengthened so that the methods are detailed enough to give the reader a complete understanding of how the study was conducted and to help guarantee the integrity of the reported results.

TABLE 6–5

Completed QUOROM Evaluation of "Treatment of Xerostomia: A Systematic Review of Therapeutic Trials"[15]

Heading	Subheading	Descriptor	Reported Y/N	Page	Article Findings
Title		Identify the report as a meta-analysis or systematic reviews of RCTs	Y	847	"Treatment of xerostomia: a systematic review of therapeutic trials."
Abstract		Use a structured format	N		No structured abstract
		Describe			
	Objectives	The clinical question explicitly			
	Data sources	The databases (i.e., list) and other information sources			
	Review methods	The selection criteria (i.e., population, intervention, outcome, and study design), methods for validity assessment, data abstraction, and study characteristics, and quantitative data synthesis in sufficient detail to permit replication.			
	Results	Characteristics of the RCTs included and excluded: qualitative and quantitative findings (i.e., point estimates and confidence intervals); and subgroup analyses			
	Conclusion	The main results			
Introduction		The explicit clinical problem, biologic rationale for the intervention, and rationale for the review	Y	847, 848	Assess the level of evidence available in therapeutic clinical trials for the management of xerostomia…Our goal is to determine the strength of the clinical trial evidence for proposed xerostomia therapies.
Methods	Searching	The information sources in detail (e.g., databases, registers, personal files, expert informants, agencies, hand-searching) and any restrictions (years considered, publication status, language of publication)	Y	848	PubMed database only, 1966–2001, RCT, human, English *Only used three search terms.*
	Selection	The inclusion and exclusion criteria (defining population, intervention, principal outcomes, and study design)	Y	848	"any therapy used for the treatment of dry mouth tested in a randomized clinical trial." No specific inclusion and exclusion criteria except population and study design.

(Continued)

TABLE 6-5

(Continued)

Heading	Subheading	Descriptor	Reported Y/N	Page	Article Findings
	Validity assessment	The criteria and process used (e.g., masked conditions, quality assessment, their findings)	Y	848	"Hadorn criteria used to evaluate each RCT…assessed 8 categories: selection of patients, allocation of patients to treatment groups, therapeutic regimen, study administration, patient withdrawals, patient blinding, blinding of outcome measures, and statistical analysis. Each bias was then classified into major and minor flaws….
	Data abstraction	The process or process used (e.g., completed independently, in duplicate)	Y	848	Two reviewers assessed each article. Discrepancies were resolved by a consensus meeting of reviewers.
	Study characteristics	The type of study design, participants' characteristics, details of intervention, outcome definitions, and how clinical heterogeneity was assessed	N		Rated each article independently
	Quantitative data synthesis	The principal measures of effect (e.g., relative risk) method of combining results (statistical testing and confidence intervals), handling of missing data: how statistical heterogeneity was assessed; a rationale of any a priori sensitivity and subgroup analysis; and any assessment of publication bias	N	848	Quantitative ranking of major and minor flaws. *This SR merely assessed the level of evidence of xerostomia therapies rather than compared effectiveness of therapies and recommend the best based on the quality of evidence available.*
Results	Trial flow	Provide a meta-analysis profile summarizing trial flow	N		
	Study characteristics	Present descriptive data for each trial (e.g., age, sample size, intervention, dose, duration, follow-up period)	Y	849	Condition, intervention. *Sample size was recorded, but not published.*
	Quantitative data synthesis	Report agreement on the selection and validity assessment, present simple summary results (for each treatment group in each trial, for each primary outcome); present data needed to calculate effect sizes and confidence intervals in intention to treat analyses (e.g., 2 × 2 tables of counts, means and SDs, proportions)	N		*Results highlighted the major and minor flaws of the RCTs selected and used SD to rate these based on Hadorn criteria. However, no simple summary of each trial—only major and minor flaws were stated.*
Discussion		Summarize key findings: discuss clinical inferences based on internal and external validity; interpret the results in light of the totality of available evidence; describe potential biases in the review process (e.g., publication bias); and suggest a future research agenda	Y	851–852	*Four Level A studies and five Level B studies were summarized. Emphasis on minimizing bias in clinical studies and better trial design is mentioned on p. 853*

96

QUOROM Statement Checklist http://www.consort-statement.org

TABLE 6–6

CONSORT Checklist for "The Efficacy of Pilocarpine and Bethanechol Upon Saliva Production in Cancer Patients with Hyposalivation Following Radiation Therapy"[16]

Paper Section and Topic	Item	Description	Reported on Page No.
Title and abstract	1	How participants were allocated to interventions (e.g., "random allocation," "randomized," "randomly assigned").	191 Randomized crossover study; however, no other details
Introduction Background	2	Scientific background and explanation of rationale.	190, 191
Methods Participants	3	Eligibility criteria for participants and the settings and locations where the data were collected.	191 Vague; no location information
Interventions	4	Precise details of the interventions intended for each group and how and when they were actually administered.	191 Precision missing (e.g., actual dosage because there were options)
Objectives	5	Specific objectives and hypotheses.	191 Purpose only
Outcomes	6	Clearly defined primary and secondary outcome measures and, when applicable, any methods used to enhance the quality of measurements (e.g., multiple observations, training of assessors).	191, 192 WSS and WRS collected same time of day
Sample size	7	How sample size was determined and, when applicable, explanation of any interim analyses and stopping rules.	191 Not clear on how sample size was determined
Randomization— sequence generation	8	Method used to generate the random allocation sequence, including details of any restrictions (e.g., blocking, stratification)	Crossover design Not stated
Randomization— allocation concealment	9	Method used to implement the random allocation sequence (e.g., numbered containers, central telephone), clarifying whether the sequence was concealed until interventions were assigned.	Not stated
Randomization— implementation	10	Who generated the allocation sequence, who enrolled participants, and who assigned participants to their groups.	Not stated
Blinding (masking)	11	Whether or not participants, those administering the interventions, and those assessing the outcomes were blinded to group assignment. When relevant, how the success of blinding was evaluated.	Not stated
Statistical methods	12	Statistical methods used to compare groups for primary outcome(s); methods for additional analyses, such as subgroup analyses and adjusted analyses.	191 Wilcoxon's rank sum test and Fisher's exact test
Results Participant flow	13	Flow of participants through each stage (a diagram is strongly recommended). Specifically, for each group report the numbers of participants randomly assigned, receiving intended treatment, completing the study protocol, and analyzed for the primary outcome. Describe protocol deviations from study as planned, together with reasons.	No flow diagram 192, 193 Tables III, IV
Recruitment	14	Dates defining the periods of recruitment and follow-up.	Not stated

(Continued)

TABLE 6-6

(Continued)

Paper Section and Topic	Item	Description	Reported on Page No.
Baseline data	15	Baseline demographic and clinical characteristics of each group.	191, 192
Numbers analyzed	16	Number of participants (denominator) in each group included in each analysis and whether the analysis was by "intention-to-treat." State the results in absolute numbers when feasible (e.g., 10/20, not 50%).	192, 193
Outcomes and estimation	17	For each primary and secondary outcome, a summary of results for each group, and the estimated effect size and its precision (e.g., 95% confidence interval).	193 No confidence interval reported
Ancillary analyses	18	Address multiplicity by reporting any other analyses performed, including subgroup analyses and adjusted analyses, indicating those prespecified and those exploratory.	192, 193
Adverse events	19	All important adverse events or side effects in each intervention group.	192, 194
Discussion Interpretation	20	Interpretation of the results, taking into account study hypotheses, sources of potential bias or imprecision and the dangers associated with multiplicity of analyses and outcomes.	194
Generalizability	21	Generalizability (external validity) of the trial findings.	194
Overall evidence	22	General interpretation of the results in the context of current evidence.	193–195

http://www.consort–statement.org

CONCLUSION

This section outlined the third step of the evidence-based decision-making (EBDM) approach—critical appraisal of the evidence to determine its validity and relevance to the patient problem. To successfully complete this step, it is important to understand research design and how the different methodologies relate to the questions being asked. To assist with the process, tools to critically appraise studies have been developed by evidence-based groups. These tools consist of a structured series of questions that help determine the validity by exploring the strengths and weaknesses of how a study was conducted, or of how information was collected, and how useful and applicable the evidence is to the specific patient problem or question being asked.

REFERENCES

1. Evidence-based Medicine Working Group. *Users' Guides to the Medical Literature, A Manual for EB Clinical Practice.* Chicago: AMA Press, 2002.
2. Critical Appraisal Skills Programme. 10 Questions to help make sense of the literature. CASP Institute of Health Sciences Web site, 2001. www.phru.nhs.uk/casp/critical_appraisal_tools.htm. Accessed April 7, 2007.
3. Centre for Evidence-Based Medicine. Critical Appraisal. Centre for Evidence-Based Medicine Web site. 2005. www.cebm.net/critical_appraisal.asp. Accessed April 7, 2007.
4. Moher D, Schulz K, Altman D, et al. The CONSORT Statement: revised recommendations for improving the quality of reports of parallel group randomized trials. *Lancet.* 2001;357:1191–1194.
5. Sackett D, Straus S, Richardson W. *Evidence-Based Medicine: How to Practice & Teach EBM.* 2nd ed. London, UK: Churchill Livingstone, 2000.
6. Evidence-based Medicine Working Group. Users' Guides to the Medical Literature, A Manual for EB Clinical Practice. Chicago: AMA, 2002. Accessed online, 4-7-07, http://www.cche.net/usersguides/therapy.asp and http://www.cche.net/usersguides/overview.asp
7. Gotrick B, Akerman S, Ericson D, Torstenson R, Tobin G. Oral pilocarpine for treatment of opioid-induced oral dryness in healthy adults. *J Dental Res.* 2004;83:393–397.
8. Moher D, Pham B, Jones A, et al. Does quality of reports of randomized trials affect estimates of intervention efficacy reported in meta-analyses? *Lancet.* 1998;352:609–613.
9. MacLehose R, Reeves B, Harvey I, et al. A systematic review of comparisons of effect sizes derived from randomised and non-randomised studies. *Health Technol Assess.* 2000;4:1–154.

10. Hulley S, Grady D, Bush T, Furberg C, et al. Randomized trial of estrogen plus progestin for secondary prevention of coronary heart disease in postmenopausal women. Heart and Estrogen/progestin Replacement Study (HERS) Research Group. *JAMA.* 1998;280:605–613.

11. Moher D, Cook D, Eastwood S, et al. Improving the quality of reports of meta-analyses of randomised controlled trials: the QUOROM statement. *Lancet.* 1999;354:1896–1900.

12. Porter S, Scully C, Hegarty A. An update of the etiology and management of xerostomia. *Oral Surg Oral Med Oral Pathol Oral Radiol Endod.* 2004;97:28–46.

13. Bossuyt P, Reitsma J, Bruns D, et al. The STARD Statement for reporting studies of diagnostic accuracy: explanation and elaboration. *Clin Chem.* 2003;49:7–18.

14. Stroup D, Berlin J, Morton S, Olkin I, et al. Meta-analysis of observational studies in epidemiology, a proposal for reporting. *JAMA.* 2000;283:2008–2012.

15. Brennan M, Shariff G, Lockhart P, Fox P. Treatment of xerostomia: a systematic review of therapeutic trials. *Dent Clin North Am.* 2002;46:847–856.

16. Gorsky M, Epstein JB, Parry J, et al. The efficacy of pilocarpine and bethanechol upon saliva production in cancer patients with hyposalivation following radiation therapy. *Oral Surg Oral Med Oral Pathol Oral Radiol Endod.* 2004;97:190–195.

SUGGESTED ACTIVITIES

At this time, complete the quiz. Next, answer the critical thinking questions. Then complete Exercise 6-1, which asks you to critique articles related to each case using the appropriate evaluation tools depending on the study design and question. Summarize the results of your appraisal in Part D of the EBDM worksheet.

QUIZ

1. Identify the three key questions in the critical appraisal process.

   a. _____

   b. _____

   c. _____

2. Describe why each of these aspects of research can influence bias.

   Source of funding _____

   _____

   Allocation of treatment groups _____

   _____

   Study sample size _____

   _____

3. Which of the guidelines consist of a structured series of yes/no questions?
   CASP
   CONSORT
   QUOROM
   STARD
   MOOSE

4. Match these guidelines with the type of study they critique.

Guideline	Type of study
CONSORT	Diagnostic study
QUOROM	Observational study
STARD	Randomized controlled trial
MOOSE	Systematic review

5. Discuss two reasons for evaluating the type of studies included in a systematic review.

   a. _____

   _____

   b. _____

   _____

6. Describe why the inclusion and exclusion criteria are important aspects of reporting the methods for a systematic review.

_____

_____

_____

7. Discuss the potential danger in basing clinical treatment decisions on observational studies.

_____

_____

_____

CRITICAL THINKING QUESTIONS

1. Compare and contrast a CASP critical appraisal form with CONSORT or QUOROM.

_____

_____

_____

_____

_____

_____

_____

2. Discuss the importance of recognizing bias in appraising the evidence.

_____

_____

_____

_____

_____

_____

_____

3. Explain why publication guidelines improve the quality of research.

_____

_____

_____

_____

_____

_____

_____

EXERCISE 6-1

Use the articles that you identified in Exercise 5-1 for each case. Using the appropriate evaluation tools (CASP, CONSORT, QUOROM, STARD, or MOOSE) appraise the evidence. Summarize the results of your appraisal in Part D of the EBDM worksheet. Attach the evaluation tool to this exercise.

Morty

Mr. Morty Kramer, a 55-year-old man, has been using unwaxed floss his whole life and flosses frequently. At his last dental appointment, he was treated by a new hygienist, who told him that he needed to change to using a waxed floss because it is more effective in removing plaque. Morty is happy with his current oral hygiene regimen and asks if he really needs to change.

Trevor

Trevor is a 27-year-old bartender who has used chewing tobacco for 13 years. He is a frequent user who chews almost 5 hours a day. He has just learned from his oral health care provider that he has developed precancerous lesions in the vestibular area where he holds the tobacco plug. This new information has motivated him to quit. Trevor knows he cannot quit by willpower alone because he has tried in the past. He wants to know if a non-nicotine aid in tobacco cessation is helpful in this endeavor, or if a nicotine patch is better in helping users permanently quit. He would like to know if behavioral therapy/counseling might help.

Dr. Bailer

Dr. Bailer recently graduated from dental school and is building a new dental practice. As he designs his building, he is trying to decide whether to purchase digital radiograph equipment or to use traditional radiography. He is interested in knowing the most accurate method for caries detection.

Jennifer

Your morning patient, Mrs. Jennifer Morris, comes to you distressed because of an article she read on the Internet about the dangers of mercury in her amalgam restorations. She is worried that her seven amalgam fillings are poisoning her. She is very concerned not only for her own health, but for her two young daughters that also have amalgam restorations. Jennifer doesn't want to replace her fillings if it isn't necessary, but needs proof that she and her children are going to be healthy.

   To reassure your patient, you give her advice based on your clinical experience and judgment; however, she still seems very upset and troubled. You inform her that you will do a thorough search of the current scientific literature and get back to her with your findings. She seems more relaxed with this thought and leaves eager to hear from you soon.

Sam

Sam is a 49-year-old man with moderate periodontitis, who was recently diagnosed with type 2 diabetes mellitus. Sam's glycosylated hemoglobin (HbA1) is 12%, which places him in the category of poorly controlled diabetes. Sam is worried that his diabetes will increase his chance of losing his teeth. He wants to know the effect and impact diabetes now has on his oral health.

Name_____ Topic_____

EBDM Worksheet PART D

Skill 3. Critically Appraising the Evidence for Its Validity and Usefulness

1. Summarize the results of the evidence that you found for your patient.

Article Reference #1:			
Type of study:	Level of evidence:	Does this answer my question? YES NO	Will I use this for my patient? YES NO
A. Are the results of the trial valid?			
B. What are the results?			
C. Will the results help my patients?			

Article Reference #2:			
Type of study:	Level of evidence:	Does this answer my question? YES NO	Will I use this for my patient? YES NO
A. Are the results of the trial valid?			
B. What are the results?			
C. Will the results help my patients?			

Article Reference #3:			
Type of study:	Level of evidence:	Does this answer my question? YES NO	Will I use this for my patient? YES NO
A. Are the results of the trial valid?			
B. What are the results?			
C. Will the results help my patients?			

Article Reference #4:			
Type of study:	Level of evidence:	Does this answer my question? YES NO	Will I use this for my patient? YES NO
A. Are the results of the trial valid?			
B. What are the results?			
C. Will the results help my patients?			

Article Reference #5:			
Type of study:	Level of evidence:	Does this answer my question? YES NO	Will I use this for my patient? YES NO
A. Are the results of the trial valid?			
B. What are the results?			
C. Will the results help my patients?			

APPENDIX

STARD Checklist of Items to Improve the Reporting of Studies on Diagnostic Accuracy

Section and Topic	Item	Describe	Reported on Page No.
Title/abstract/ keywords	1	The article as a study on diagnostic accuracy (recommend MeSH heading 'sensitivity and specificity')	
Introduction	2	The research question(s), such as estimating diagnostic accuracy or comparing accuracy between tests or across participant groups	
		Methods	
Participants	3	The study population: the inclusion and exclusion criteria, setting(s) and location(s) where the data were collected	
	4	Participant recruitment: was this based on presenting symptoms, results from previous tests, or the fact that the participants had received the index test(s) or the reference standard?	
	5	Participant sampling: was this a consecutive series of patients defined by selection criteria in (3) and (4)? If not specify how patients were further selected.	
	6	Data collection: were the participants identified and data collected before the index test(s) and reference standards were performed (prospective study) or after (retrospective study)?	
Reference standard	7	The reference standard and its rationale	
Test methods	8	Technical specification of material and methods involved including how and when measurements were taken, and/or cite references for index test(s) and reference standard	
	9	Definition and rationale for the units, cutoffs, or categories of the results of the index test(s) and the reference standard	
	10	The number, training and expertise of the persons (a) executing and (b) reading the index test(s) and the reference standard	

(Continued)

Section and Topic	Item	Describe	Reported on Page No.
	11	Whether or not the reader(s) of the index test(s) and reference standard were blinded (masked) to the results of the other test(s) and describe any information available to them	
Statistical methods	12	Methods for calculating measures of diagnostic accuracy or making comparisons, and the statistical methods used to quantify uncertainty (e.g., 95% confidence intervals)	
	13	Methods for calculating test reproducibility, if done	
		Results	
Participants	14	When study was done, including beginning and ending dates of recruitment	
	15	Clinical and demographic characteristics (e.g., age, sex, spectrum of presenting symptoms, comorbidity, current treatments, recruitment center)	
	16	How many participants satisfying the criteria for inclusion did or did not undergo the index test or the reference standard? Describe why participants failed to receive either test (a flow diagram is strongly recommended)	
Reference standard	17	Time interval and any treatment administered between index and reference standard	
	18	Distribution of severity of disease (define criteria) in those with the target condition; describe other diagnoses in participants without the target condition	
Test results	19	A cross-tabulation of the results of the index test(s) by the results of the reference standard; for continuous results, the distribution of the test results by the results of the reference standard	
	20	Indeterminate results, missing responses and outliers of index test(s) stratified by reference standard result and how they were handled	
	21	Adverse events of index test(s) and reference standard	
Estimation	22	Estimates of diagnostic accuracy and measures of statistical uncertainty (e.g., 95% confidence intervals)	
	23	Estimates of variability of diagnostic accuracy between subgroups of participants, readers, or centers, if done	
	24	Measures of test reproducibility, if done	
Discussion	25	The clinical applicability of the study findings	

To improve dissemination of the STARD statement, the STARD statement including the checklist has free copyright. Adapted from www.stard-statement.org.

A Proposed Reporting Checklist for Authors, Editors, and Reviewers of Meta-Analyses of Observational Studies (MOOSE)[14]

Reporting of background should include:

- Problem definition
- Hypothesis statement
- Description of study outcome(s)
- Type of exposure or intervention used
- Type of study designs used
- Study population

Reporting of search strategy should include:

- Qualifications of searchers (e.g., librarians, investigators)
- Search strategy, including time period included in the synthesis and keywords
- Effort to include all available studies, including contact with authors
- Databases and registries searched
- Search software used, name and version, including special features used (e.g., explosion)
- Use of hand searching (e.g., reference lists of obtained articles)
- List of citations located and those excluded, including justification
- Method of addressing articles published in languages other than English
- Method of handling abstracts and unpublished studies
- Description of any contact with authors

Reporting of methods should include:

- Description of relevance or appropriateness of studies assembled for assessing the hypothesis to be tested
- Rationale for the selection and coding of data (e.g., sound clinical principles or convenience)
- Documentation of how data were classified and coded (e.g., multiple raters, blinding, and interrater reliability)
- Assessment of confounding (e.g., comparability of cases and controls in studies where appropriate)

- Assessment of study quality, including blinding of quality assessors; stratification or regression on possible predictors of study results
- Assessment of heterogeneity
- Description of statistical methods (e.g., complete description of fixed or random effects models, justification of whether the chosen models account for predictors of study results, dose-response models, or cumulative meta-analysis) in sufficient detail to be replicated
- Provision of appropriate tables and graphics

Reporting of results should include:

- Graphic summarizing individual study estimates and overall estimate
- Table giving descriptive information for each study included
- Results of sensitivity testing (e.g., subgroup analysis)
- Indication of statistical uncertainty of findings

Reporting of discussion should include:

- Quantitative assessment of bias (e.g., publication bias)
- Justification for exclusion (e.g., exclusion of non–English-language citations)
- Assessment of quality of included studies

Reporting of conclusions should include:

- Consideration of alternative explanations for observed results
- Generalization of the conclusions (i.e., appropriate for the data presented and within the domain of the literature review)
- Guidelines for future research
- Disclosure of funding source

Adapted from www.consort-statement.org/MOOSE/moose.pdf, with permission.

CHAPTER 7

Evaluating Web-Based Health Information

Critically Appraising the Evidence for its Validity and Usefulness (Clinical Applicability).

PURPOSE

The purpose of this section is to discuss Web-based health information as it relates to patient care. Internet Web sites are often the first place students and patients look for information, often using a Web browser such as Google. This section will discuss three types of Web-based health resources including government, university, and industry Web sites. In addition to providing valuable Web resources, this section will outline several key factors to consider when evaluating Web-based resources to eliminate bias.

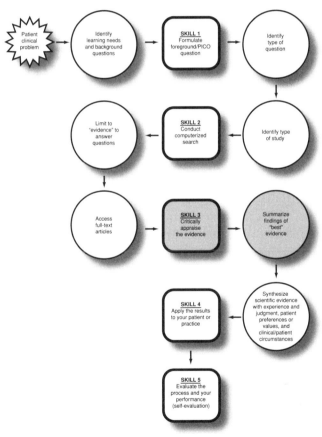

OBJECTIVES

After completing this chapter, readers will be able to:

1. Identify the Internet domain of Web-based resources.
2. Evaluate Web-based resources.

SUGGESTED ACTIVITIES

Quiz
Critical Thinking Questions
Exercise 7-1

The Internet, or World Wide Web (WWW), has revolutionized how information is accessed, shared, and communicated. The number of people with Internet access continues to grow at an extremely rapid pace. More than 70% of Americans have access to the Internet.[1] In 2000, 52 million Americans sought information about health care online and 47% said the information they found influenced their decisions.[2] In a study conducted by the Pew Internet Project in March of 2002, 62% of Americans sought health care information online.[3] As the Web becomes an integral part of people's everyday lives for buying products and finding information, there is a growing need to distinguish the credibility of Web sites.[1]

WEB-BASED HEALTH RESOURCES

There are three main types of Web-based health resources—government, university, and industry Web sites—that include professional organizations, public or private companies, and individual dentist/doctor Web sites that are usually associated with their practices. Every Web site has a unique address or URL (unified resource locator). The URL endings often describe the domain or what type of provider is hosting the Web site (Table 7-1).

EVALUATING INTERNET SOURCES

As discussed in Chapter 1, patients come to their appointments educated (sometimes inaccurately) about new dental products, treatment procedures, and diagnostic tests they have learned about through advertisements and the Internet. However, many of the resources available to the general public are biased, inaccurate, or not appropriate for the patient. It is important for practitioners to develop the skills to analyze and evaluate these sources to accurately address patient's concerns with valid evidence. The ability to do this while integrating good science with clinical judgment enhances

TABLE 7–1

Internet Domains

Type of Provider	URL Endings
Nonprofit organizations (can now be anyone regardless of the nature of the site)	.org
Commercial companies and for-profit organizations, individual dentist/doctor Web sites (can now be anyone regardless of the nature of the site)	.com
Network access groups (can now be anyone regardless of the nature of the site)	.net
Federal government	.gov
Military agencies and organizations	.mil
Educational organizations granting degrees	.edu

credibility, builds trust and confidence with the patient, and may enhance the patient's quality of care.

In a research report that studied how people evaluate a site's credibility, participants made decisions about the people or organization behind the site based mostly on the site's overall visual appeal. Nearly half of the 26,448 consumers that participated (46.1% overall and 41.8% relative to health sites) linked credibility to visual aspects of the site including layout, typography, font size, and color schemes rather than content, sources, depth, and quality of information.[4]

Currency and Credibility

It is often difficult to distinguish between an authoritative source and a site that is essentially an advertisement or an opinion. The Medical Library Association recommends that Internet users review a health Web site to determine sponsorships of both commercial and noncommercial groups that have contributed funding, services, or material to the site and to verify that information is current and factual (verifiable from a primary information source) or clearly stated as an opinion, and the information is appropriate for the audience (i.e., health care provider or consumer).[5] This is important because there are many health sites that contain inaccurate or misleading information or are written by individuals without the appropriate credentials. Information should be referenced to published information and should be authored by credentialed professionals with the authority to discuss the topic matter.

Identifying Bias

The same criteria used in identifying bias published research outlined in Chapter 6 are also applicable when evaluating Web sites. It is important to review the information to determine if the site is funded by an entity that may benefit from the consumer reading or ac-

cessing the information that can cause bias in the way information is presented. Consumer WebWatch guidelines state that sites should clearly disclose their ownership, private or public, naming their parent company and should clearly distinguish advertising from news and information. This includes "in-house" advertising or cross-corporate ad sponsorships. In addition, sites should clearly disclose relevant business relationships, including sponsored links to other sites. For example, a site that directs a reader to another site to purchase something should clearly disclose any financial relationship between the two sites. Sites should also identify sponsors in text or on an "About Us" page.

Evaluation Checklists

There are several checklists and resources that are available that prompt key questions to answer and are helpful when evaluating Internet resources. These URLs are listed in Table 7-2 under Web Site Evaluation. *Evaluation Criteria* by Susan Beck at New Mexico State University has a series of questions based on the topics of authority, objectivity, currency, and coverage. *Thinking Critically about World Wide Web Resources* by Esther Grassian at UCLA provides a list of key questions based on the topics of content and evaluation, source and date, and structure. In addition, Consumer WebWatch, a grant-funded project of Consumers Union, the nonprofit publisher of *Consumer Reports* magazine and ConsumerReports.org, has published guidelines that promote Web site credibility regarding identity, advertising and sponsorships, customer services, correctness, and privacy. To date, more than 250 major Web sites have pledged their compliance to those guidelines. Figure 7-1 is an evaluation checklist that incorporates a collaboration of key questions that are important to consider when determining the credibility of health care information on the Web.

TABLE 7–2

Evidence-Based Decision-Making Resources

Point-of-Care Resources

Clinical evidence	www.clinicalevidence.com
Evidence based on call	www.eboncall.org/
Evidence Watch	http://evidencewatch.com/
First Consult	www.firstconsult.com
InfoPOEMS and InfoRetriever	www.infopoems.com/
Family Physicians Inquiries Network	www.fpin.org/
UpToDate	www.uptodate.com/
The Trip Database searches more than 61 sites of high-quality medical information on the Web	www.tripdatabase.com/
Combined Health Information Database (CHID)	http://chid.nih.gov/
Netting the evidence access to helpful organizations and useful learning resources	www.shef.ac.uk/~scharr/ir/netting
Drug databases • Corey Nahman.com updated daily • RxList • MEDLINEplus Health Information	 www.coreynahman.com/druginfopage.html www.rxlist.com/ www.nlm.nih.gov/medlineplus/druginformation.html
Lexi-Comp	http://store.lexi.com/web/index.jsp
Google Scholar	http://scholar.google.com/

Web Site Evaluation Sites

Consumer WebWatch	www.consumerwebwatch.org/consumer-reports-webwatch-guidelines.cfm
Evaluation Criteria from The Good, The Bad, and The Ugly: or, Why It's a Good Idea to Evaluate Web Sources	http://lib.nmsu.edu/instruction/evalcrit.html
Thinking Critically about World Wide Web Resources, by Esther Grassian, UCLA College Library	www.library.ucla.edu/libraries/college/help/critical/index.htm
The Medical Library Associations: A User's Guide to Finding and Evaluating Health Information on the Web	www.mlanet.org/resources/userguide.html#3
Health on the Net Foundation	www.hon.ch/index.html

Evidence-Based Databases and Publications

PubMed—Free public version of Medline	http://pubmed.gov
SUMSearch—a "meta-search" engine for evidence-based medicine resources University of Texas Health Science Center at San Antonio	http://SUMSearch.uthscsa.edu
Cochrane Collaboration	www.cochrane.de/
Cochrane Oral Health Group Abstracts of Systematic Reviews	www.cochrane-oral.man.ac.uk/abstracts.htm
DARE (Database of Abstracts of Reviews of Effectiveness)	http://nhscrd.york.ac.uk/darehp.htm
DARE listing of Dental systematic reviews	www.cochrane-oral.man.ac.uk/dental_systematic_reviews.htm
Bandolier—Dental and Oral Health	www.jr2.ox.ac.uk/bandolier/booth/booths/dental.html
Evidence-Based Dentistry journal	www.nature.com/ebd/index.html
Journal of Evidence-based Dental Practice	www.us.elsevierhealth.com/product.jsp?isbn=15323382
ADA guidelines	www.ada.org/prof/resources/positions/statements/index.asp

(Continued)

TABLE 7-2

(Continued)

National Guideline Clearinghouse	www.guideline.gov
Evidence-Based Tutorials	
Evidence-based clinical practice	www.urmc.rochester.edu/hslt/miner/resources/evidence_based/index.cfm
Introduction to EBM, Duke University/UNC	www.hsl.unc.edu/services/tutorials/ebm/index.htm
SUNY Health Sciences evidence-based medicine course from SUNY Downstate Medical Center	http://servers.medlib.hscbklyn.edu/ebm/toc.html
PubMed tutorial, National Library of Medicine	www.nlm.nih.gov/bsd/pubmed_tutorial/m1001.html
Purdue University evaluating Internet sources and sites: a tutorial	www.lib.purdue.edu/ugrl/staff/sharkey/interneteval/
Research Design and Statistical Terms and Concepts	
Guide to Research Methods, The Evidence Pyramid	http://servers.medlib.hscbklyn.edu/ebm/2100.htm
Critical Appraisal Skills Programme (CASP)	www.phru.nhs.uk/casp/critical_appraisal_tools.htm
Evidence-Based Centers	
Agency for Healthcare Research and Quality (AHRQ)	www.ahrq.gov/
Centre for Evidence-based Dentistry	www.cebd.org
Centre for Evidence Based Medicine	www.cebm.net
Center for Evidence Based Medicine—University of Toronto	www.cebm.utoronto.ca
Centres for Health Evidence	www.cche.net
The Cochrane Collaboration	www.cochrane.org
Evidence-Based Informatics, HIRU at McMaster	http://hiru.mcmaster.ca/
Evidence Based Decision Making, National Center for Dental Hygiene Research	www.usc.edu/ebnet

POINT OF CARE TOOLS AND ONLINE RESOURCES FOR EVIDENCE-BASED DECISION MAKING

There are many resources for using and applying evidence-based decision making (EBDM). As technology advances and the need to access information at the point of care increases, manufacturers are responding to those needs. In addition to small books and drug indexes, hand-held devices with networking, computing, telephone/fax, and Internet features, commonly known as personal digital assistants (PDAs) are becoming an integral tool at the point of care. PDAs function as a personal organizer, cellular phone, fax, e-mail, and Internet connection and can hold vast amounts of evidence that can be used when treating patients. Many Web sites provide PDA downloads to access databases, articles, drug information, EB calculators (programs that aid in calculating evidence-based numbers [i.e., NNT]), and publications. A list of key EBDM resources, including Point of Care URLs, is outlined in Table 7-2. Because Web links change over time,

please refer to the EBDM Web site at www.usc.edu/ebnet for current links.

The Medical Library Association has published their Ten Most Useful Consumer Health Websites[5] that may provide a good foundation for finding health related information for your patients. These are summarized here.

Cancer.gov (www.cancer.gov/) is the official Web site for The National Cancer Institute (NCI), a component of the National Institutes of Health (NIH), one of eight agencies that compose the Public Health Service (PHS) in the Department of Health and Human Services (DHHS). The NCI, established under the National Cancer Act of 1937, is the federal government's principal agency for cancer research and training. NCI coordinates the National Cancer Program, which conducts and supports research, training, health information dissemination, and other programs with respect to the cause, diagnosis, prevention, and treatment of cancer, rehabilitation from cancer, and the continuing care of cancer patients and the families of cancer patients.

Name_____Topic_____

EBDM Worksheet Part E
Evaluating the Web sites where information
pertinent to the patient is found.

Skill 3. Critically Appraising the Evidence for its Validity and Usefulness

	URL of page evaluated: http://	URL of page evaluated: http://
Information about the site		
Domain	❑ .com, .org, .net ❑ .edu ❑ .mil/.gov/ ❑ other:_____	❑ .com, .org, .net ❑ .edu ❑ .mil/.gov/ ❑ other:_____
Is the domain appropriate for the content?	❑ Yes ❑ No	❑ Yes ❑ No
Is the purpose and mission of the Web site appropriate for the information posted?	❑ Yes ❑ No	❑ Yes ❑ No
Ownership	❑ Private:_____ ❑ Public:_____	❑ Private:_____ ❑ Public:_____
Webmaster contact info	**Name:** **Address:** **Email:**	**Name:** **Address:** **Email:**
Date information was posted	**mm/dd/yr**	**mm/dd/yr**
Date site was last updated	**mm/dd/yr**	**mm/dd/yr**
Credibility of information		
Is the information current?	❑ Yes ❑ No	❑ Yes ❑ No
Is it clear who wrote the page/information?	**Name:** **Email:** **Credentials:**	**Name:** **Email:** **Credentials:**
Is the writer qualified to discuss the topic?	❑ Yes ❑ No	❑ Yes ❑ No
Is there bias, opinions?	❑ Yes ❑ No	❑ Yes ❑ No
Is the information referenced, reliable, and accurate from print/published research?	❑ Yes ❑ No Describe your answer:	❑ Yes ❑ No Describe your answer:
Are the sources current and well-documented?	❑ Yes ❑ No	❑ Yes ❑ No
Are there links to more resources?	❑ Yes ❑ No	❑ Yes ❑ No
What is the purpose of the information? Check all that apply.	❑ **Inform** ❑ **Explain** ❑ **Persuade** ❑ **Disclose** ❑ **Sell** ❑ **Advertise**	❑ **Inform** ❑ **Explain** ❑ **Persuade** ❑ **Disclose** ❑ **Sell** ❑ **Advertise**
Sponsorship		
Is a sponsor clearly identified?	❑ Yes ❑ No	❑ Yes ❑ No
Is there an Advisory board or consultants?	❑ Yes ❑ No	❑ Yes ❑ No
Are the partnerships or advertisements clear?	❑ Yes ❑ No	❑ Yes ❑ No
Is the information usable based on the above?	❑ **Yes** ❑ **No**	❑ **Yes** ❑ **No**

FIGURE 7–1   Evaluating a health Web site checklist (Part E of the EBDM Worksheet).

Centers for Disease Control and Prevention (www.cdc. gov/), an agency of the Department of Health and Human Services, is dedicated to promoting "health and quality of life by preventing and controlling disease, injury, and disability." Of special interest to the consumer are the resources about diseases, conditions, and other special topics arranged under "Health Topics A-Z," and "Travelers' Health," with health recommendations for travelers worldwide. There are also sections on health topics in the news and health hoaxes. Information is also available in Spanish.

familydoctor.org (http://familydoctor.org/) is operated by the American Academy of Family Physicians (AAFP), a national medical organization representing more than 93,700 family physicians, family practice residents, and medical students. All of the information on this site has been written and reviewed by physicians and patient education professionals at the AAFP.

Healthfinder (www.healthfinder.gov/) is a gateway consumer health information Web site whose goal is "to improve consumer access to selected health information from government agencies, their many partner organizations, and other reliable sources that serve the public interest." Menu lists on its home page provide links to online journals, medical dictionaries, minority health, and prevention and self-care. The developer and sponsor of this site is the Office of Disease Prevention and Health Promotion, Department of Health and Human Services, with other agencies that also can be linked to via the site. Access to resources on the site is also available in Spanish.

HIV InSite (http://hivinsite.ucsf.edu/) is a project of the University of California San Francisco AIDS Research Institute. Designed as a gateway to in-depth information about particular aspects of HIV/AIDS, it provides numerous links to many authoritative sources. Subjects are arranged into key topics and the site may also be searched by key words. Many items are provided in full text, and information is available in English and Spanish.

Kidshealth (www.kidshealth.org/) provides doctor-approved health information about children from before birth through adolescence. Created by The Nemours Foundation's Center for Children's Health Media, KidsHealth provides families with accurate, up-to-date, and jargon-free health information they can use. KidsHealth has been on the Web since 1995 and has been accessed by more than 170 million visitors.

MayoClinic (www.mayoclinic.com/) is an extension of the Mayo Clinic's commitment to provide health education to patients and the general public. Editors of the site include more than 2,000 physicians, scientists, writers, and educators at the Mayo Clinic, a nonprofit institution with more than 100 years of history in patient care, medical research, and education. The Web site has added interactive tools to assist consumers in managing their health. This site supersedes the previous site, Mayo Clinic Health Oasis.

Medem (http://medem.com/) is a project of the leading medical societies in the United States. Some of the founding societies include the American Medical Association, the American Academy of Pediatrics, and the American College of Obstetricians and Gynecologists. The site was developed to provide "a trusted online source for credible, comprehensive, and clinical healthcare information, and secure, confidential communications." The Medical Library is divided into four major categories: life stages, diseases and conditions, therapies and health strategies, and health and society.

MEDLINEplus (http://medlineplus.gov/) is a consumer-oriented Web site established by the National Library of Medicine, the world's largest biomedical library and creator of the MEDLINE database. An alphabetical list of health topics consists of more than 300 specific diseases, conditions, and wellness issues. Each Health topic page contains links to authoritative information on that subject, as well as an optional link to a preformulated MEDLINE search that provides journal article citations on the subject. Additional resources include physician and hospital directories, several online medical dictionaries, and consumer drug information available by generic or brand name.

NOAH: New York Online Access to Health (www.noah-health.org/) is a unique collection of state, local, and federal health resources for consumers. NOAH's mission is "to provide high quality, full text information for consumers that is accurate, timely, relevant, and unbiased." Information is arranged in alphabetical health topics, which are then narrowed to include definitions, care and treatment, and lists of information resources. Information is available in both English and Spanish, and the majority of items are provided in full text.

CONCLUSION

There are many useful Internet sites that provide information about health-related topics. Lifelong learners should have the skills to appraise the evidence found on the Internet before incorporating it into the EBDM process. Understanding the types of Web-based health resources and Internet domains is useful in identifying the source of information. Having the skills to evaluate the currency and accuracy of the information, the credibility of the authors, and any bias ensures that practitioner's accurately address patient's concerns with valid evidence.

REFERENCES

1. Nielsen//NetRatings (NNR 3/2004), www.nielsennetratings.com

2. Palmer, PR. Oral health care finds its niche, online. *Access.* 2001; 15:20–29.

3. Rainie L, Packel D. More online, *Doing More: 16 Million Newcomers Gain Internet Access in the Last Half of 2000 as Women, Minorities, and Families with Modest Incomes Continue to Surge Online.* Issued February 18, 2001. Washington DC: The Pew Internet and American Life Project tracking report.

4. Fogg BJ, Soohoo C, Danielson DR, et al. How do users evaluate the credibility of Web sites? A study with over 2,500 participants. DUX '03: Proceedings of the 2003 conference on designing for user experiences, 2003. ACM Portal Web site. http://doi.acm.org/10.1145/997078.997097. Accessed January 16, 2008.

5. Medical Library Association. A user's guide to finding and evaluating health information on the Web. www.mlanet.org/resources/userguide.html#3. Accessed January 16, 2008.

SUGGESTED ACTIVITIES

At this time, complete the quiz. Next, complete the critical thinking questions. Then, work through Exercise 7-1, using the EBDM worksheet Part E to evaluate at least two Internet sites that relates to each of the five case studies and strengthen the third skill of the EBDM process: critically appraising the evidence.

QUIZ

1. In a Web site credibility study, results demonstrated that most people tend to evaluate credibility based on what?
   a. Sources
   b. Domain
   c. Color schemes
   d. Content of information

2. When determining the credibility of a Web site, it is important to review
   a. Sponsorships
   b. Typography
   c. Color schemes
   d. Layout

3. The URL is the:
   a. Unique record label
   b. Untimely restructured location
   c. Unique readable location
   d. Unified resource locator

4. The URL often describes the:
   a. domain
   b. Internet service provider
   c. the Web site host
   d. all of the above

5. There are several internet domains that can now be used by anyone regardless of the nature of the Web site. These include:
   a. .com and .org and .net
   b. .org and .net and .tv
   c. .com and .net and .tv
   d. .com and .tv and .org

CRITICAL THINKING QUESTIONS

1. Why is it important to evaluate internet resources?

_____

_____

_____

_____

_____

_____

_____

_____

_____

_____

2. Discuss why bias influences information on a Web site?

_____

_____

_____

_____

_____

_____

_____

_____

_____

_____

3. Compare and contrast two Internet resources on the same topic—one that provides very good information about the topic and one that you would not recommend. Discuss what makes the good site valuable and what would make the site that you would not recommend better.

_____

_____

_____

_____

_____

_____

_____

_____

_____

EXERCISE 7-1

Use Part E of the EBDM Worksheet to evaluate at least two Internet sites that relate to each of the five patient case scenarios.

Morty

Mr. Morty Kramer, a 55-year-old man, has been using unwaxed floss his whole life and flosses frequently. At his last dental appointment, he was treated by a new hygienist, who told him that he needed to change to using a waxed floss because it is more effective in removing plaque. Morty is happy with his current oral hygiene regimen and asks if he really needs to change.

Trevor

Trevor is a 27-year-old bartender who has used chewing tobacco for 13 years. He is a frequent user who chews almost 5 hours a day. He has just learned from his oral health care provider that he has developed precancerous lesions in the vestibular area where he holds the tobacco plug. This new information has motivated him to quit. Trevor knows he cannot quit by willpower alone because he has tried in the past. He wants to know if a non-nicotine aid in tobacco cessation is helpful in this endeavor, or if a nicotine patch is better in helping users permanently quit. He would like to know if behavioral therapy/counseling might help.

Dr. Bailer

Dr. Bailer recently graduated from dental school and is building a new dental practice. As he designs his building, he is trying to decide whether to purchase digital radiograph equipment or to use traditional radiography. He is interested in knowing the most accurate method for caries detection.

Jennifer

Your morning patient, Mrs. Jennifer Morris, comes to you distressed because of an article she read on the Internet about the dangers of mercury in her amalgam restorations. She is worried that her seven amalgam fillings are poisoning her. She is very concerned not only for her own health, but for her two young daughters that also have amalgam restorations. Jennifer doesn't want to replace her fillings if it isn't necessary, but needs proof that she and her children are going to be healthy.

To reassure your patient, you give her advice based on your clinical experience and judgment; however, she still seems very upset and troubled. You inform her that you will do a thorough search of the current scientific literature and get back to her with your findings. She seems more relaxed with this thought and leaves eager to hear from you soon.

Sam

Sam is a 49-year-old man with moderate periodontitis, who was recently diagnosed with type 2 diabetes mellitus. Sam's glycosylated hemoglobin (HbA1) is 12%, which places him in the category of poorly controlled diabetes. Sam is worried that his diabetes will increase his chance of losing his teeth. He wants to know the effect and impact diabetes now has on his oral health.

Name_____Topic_____

EBDM Worksheet Part E
Evaluating the Web sites where information
pertinent to the patient is found.

Skill 3. Critically Appraising the Evidence for its Validity and Usefulness

	URL of page evaluated: http://	URL of page evaluated: http://
Information about the site		
Domain	❑ .com, .org, .net ❑ .edu ❑ .mil/.gov/ ❑ other:_____	❑ .com, .org, .net ❑ .edu ❑ .mil/.gov/ ❑ other:_____
Is the domain appropriate for the content?	❑ Yes ❑ No	❑ Yes ❑ No
Is the purpose and mission of the Web site appropriate for the information posted?	❑ Yes ❑ No	❑ Yes ❑ No
Ownership	❑ Private:_____ ❑ Public:_____	❑ Private:_____ ❑ Public:_____
Webmaster contact info	Name: Address: Email:	Name: Address: Email:
Date information was posted	mm/dd/yr	mm/dd/yr
Date site was last updated	mm/dd/yr	mm/dd/yr
Credibility of Information		
Is the information current?	❑ Yes ❑ No	❑ Yes ❑ No
Is it clear who wrote the page/information?	Name: Email: Credentials:	Name: Email: Credentials:
Is the writer qualified to discuss the topic?	❑ Yes ❑ No	❑ Yes ❑ No
Is there bias, opinions?	❑ Yes ❑ No	❑ Yes ❑ No
Is the information referenced, reliable, and accurate from print/published research?	❑ Yes ❑ No Describe your answer:	❑ Yes ❑ No Describe your answer:
Are the sources current and well-documented?	❑ Yes ❑ No	❑ Yes ❑ No
Are there links to more resources?	❑ Yes ❑ No	❑ Yes ❑ No
What is the purpose of the information? Check all that apply.	❑ Inform ❑ Explain ❑ Persuade ❑ Disclose ❑ Sell ❑ Advertise	❑ Inform ❑ Explain ❑ Persuade ❑ Disclose ❑ Sell ❑ Advertise
Sponsorship		
Is a sponsor clearly identified?	❑ Yes ❑ No	❑ Yes ❑ No
Is there an Advisory board or consultants?	❑ Yes ❑ No	❑ Yes ❑ No
Are the partnerships or advertisements clear?	❑ Yes ❑ No	❑ Yes ❑ No
Is the information usable based on the above?	❑ Yes ❑ No	❑ Yes ❑ No

CHAPTER 8

Applying the Evidence to Practice

SKILL 4

Applying the Results of the Appraisal, or Evidence, in Clinical Practice.

PURPOSE

The purpose of this section is to discuss the fourth step in the evidence-based decision-making (EBDM) process: applying the results of the evidence into clinical practice. This step involves understanding the type of statistical analysis needed to determine if the valid results found are important and, if so, are they feasible to implement with a patient. Understanding how to present statistical information to patients in a clear and unambiguous manner will help in making good patient care decisions. In addition, understanding the clinical significance of research findings and translation of the findings to the individual patient is an important aspect of the fourth step. Again, the case study of Gail will be used for discussion in relating the scientific evidence to patient situations.

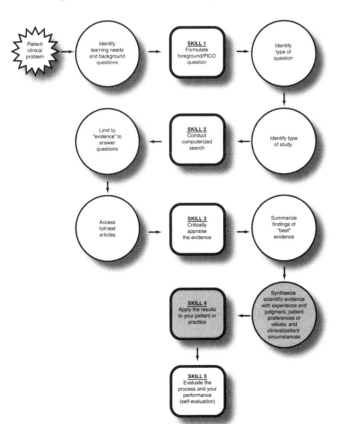

OBJECTIVES

After completing this chapter, readers will be able to:

1. Differentiate between common ways used to report outcomes.
   - Relative risk (RR) and relative risk reduction (RRR)
   - Absolute risk reduction (ARR)
   - Odds ratio (OR)
   - Numbers needed to treat (NNT)
   - Sensitivity and specificity
   - Positive predictive values (PPV) and negative predictive values (NPV)
   - Likelihood ratios
2. Explain the difference between absolute and relative difference in reporting outcomes.
3. Identify the measures used to report outcomes from studies related to therapy/prevention, prognosis, harm/etiology/causation, diagnosis, and systematic reviews.
4. Identify the difference between screening and diagnostic tests.
5. Discuss how the presentation of statistics can influence treatment decisions
   a. Distinguish between statistical and clinical significance
   b. Relate evidence to patient situations
      - Discuss research findings with Gail
      - Incorporate statistics to formulate patient recommendations

SUGGESTED ACTIVITIES

Quiz
Critical Thinking Questions
Exercise 8-1

Research findings are only a part of good clinical decision-making. As discussed in Chapter 1, EBDM is the formalized process of identifying, searching for, and interpreting the results of the best scientific evidence, which is considered in conjunction with the clinician's experience and judgment, the patient's preferences and values,

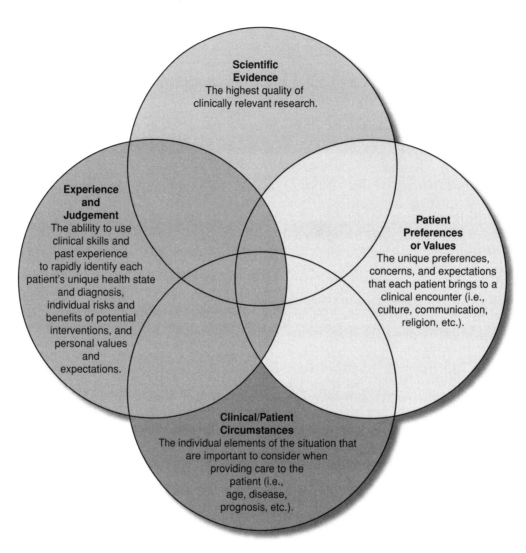

FIGURE 8-1 Evidence-based decision-making process. © 2005 Jane L. Forrest, Ed.

and the clinical/patient circumstances when making patient care decisions (Fig. 8-1). Therefore, when applying the results of the appraisal, one must also consider the other three aspects of the decision-making process.

COMMON WAYS USED TO REPORT STATISTICAL DATA AND OUTCOMES

Measures Used to Report Outcomes from Studies Related to Therapy/Prevention and Harm/Etiology/Causation

After the methods are determined to be valid, the next step is to determine if the results, potential benefits, or harms are important. This is achieved by looking at whether there is an association between specific treatments and outcomes or exposures, and the condition of interest, and then the strength of that association. Differences between groups in clinical trials are generally straightforward when expressed in terms of the mean values; whereas, results presented as *proportions*, such as relative risk reduction, absolute risk reduction, odds ratio and NNT, are more challenging to understand.[1]

ABSOLUTE AND RELATIVE DIFFERENCES

However presented, statistical data should be represented in a way that provides clear insight so that good treatment decisions can be made.[2] The following hypothetical example of the need for endodontic retreatment illustrates the difference in how statistics can be reported, which, in turn, can influence how information is presented to patients and the clinical decisions made.

Example: Endodontic Retreatment Needs

A hypothetical study was conducted to determine the success rate of endodontic treatment with success defined as preventing the need for retreatment. After 3 years, investigators found that 6.0% of the patients in the placebo group (i.e., those who received the "standard" endodontic treatment) needed retreatment, whereas only 3.0% of those in the experimental group (i.e., who received the "new" endodontic treatment) needed retreatment. The difference between these results can be represented in absolute and relative terms and each can be expressed in the following ways:[3]

Absolute difference is expressed as the arithmetic difference between rates

- 3% fewer patients in the new endodontic treatment group needed retreatment. This represents an absolute difference, *or the arithmetic difference in rates* between 6.0% and 3.0% (6% – 3%, which is equal to a 3% decrease).
- The standard endodontic treatment increases the need for retreatment for 3% more patients. Again, this represents an absolute difference, *or the arithmetic difference in rates* between 3.0% and 6.0%, which is equal to a 3% increase.

Relative difference is expressed as a proportion of patients

- The new endodontic treatment reduced the need for retreatment by 50% (i.e., the *proportion of patients* or percent increase or difference in a group in whom the event is observed); starting at 6% and going to 3% cuts the numbers of individuals needing retreatment in half.
- The standard endodontic treatment increases the need for retreatment by 100%. Again, this *proportion of patients* represents a relative difference going from 3% to 6%, doubling the number of patients—a 100% increase.

Based on the presentation of the results in absolute terms (3% reduction) or in relative terms (50% reduction), clinicians could decide to start using the "new" endodontic treatment or stop using it. Factored into this decision would be the time, cost, number of patients needing endodontic treatment in their practice, and number of visits required to determine if the outcome (achieving a 3% or 50% decrease in retreatment needs) is worthwhile.

In addition to absolute and relative differences, probabilities and risks associated with disease and exposures can be presented in additional ways based on analysis of the frequency of those who experienced a particular outcome or event in the treatment and control groups. Often, the outcome is a dichotomous event (yes or no): either it occurs or does not occur. Also, the event can be either positive (improving a poor condition) or negative (developing a disease or tooth loss).

Events that are not purely dichotomous also may be presented as though they are by establishing a threshold or degree of change that represents an important improvement or deterioration.[1] For example, an event can be defined as 30% improvement over the baseline value, so for those who experience a 30% or greater improvement, their outcome would be reported as *yes*, it "occurs."

A comparison of proportions from two independent groups is commonly expressed in a 2 × 2 contingency table, as seen in Table 8-1. From this table, several different outcomes often reported in the literature can be expressed, such as relative risk, relative risk reduction, absolute risk reduction, numbers needed to treat, and odds ratio. All of these outcomes, with the exception of OR, are used to determine if the results from a therapy/prevention trial are important. OR, along with RR, is used for studies related to harm/etiology. Also, the OR is the measure of choice in the analysis of case control studies.

Hypothetical values are inserted on Table 8-2 to demonstrate how each of these outcomes is calculated for a study examining 5-year tooth loss for 1,000 individuals after endodontic treatment comparing when a crown has been placed or not. In this hypothetical study, the experimental group is comprised of individuals who received a crown and the control group includes those individuals who did not receive a crown after endodontic therapy. The disease or condition of interest is tooth loss.

TABLE 8-1

2 × 2 Contingency Table

Exposure Treatment or Risk	Outcome Disease/Condition		Total
	Yes	*No*	*Total*
Yes	A	B	A + B
No	C	D	C + D
Total	A + C	B + D	N

TABLE 8-2

Hypothetical Data for 5-Year Tooth Loss After Endodontic Therapy

Crown Placed	Tooth Loss		Total
	Yes	*No*	*Total*
Yes Crown	50 A	600 B	650 A + B
No Crown	250 C	100 D	350 C + D
Total	300 A + C	700 B + D	1000 N

Based on this hypothetical example data, 5-year tooth loss data can be reported using the following statistics, the definitions of which are taken from the Center for Evidence-Based Medicine:[4]

1. **Event rate** is the proportion of patients in a group in whom the event is observed. Therefore, if out of 1,000 patients, the event (tooth loss) is observed in 300, the event rate is 0.30, or 30%. The **control event rate (CER)** and the **experimental event rate (EER)** are used to refer to the control and experimental groups of patients respectively and both rates are important in calculating relative and absolute differences.
   - The **CER** is the proportion of patients in the control group (those who did not receive a crown) who experience the event (i.e., tooth loss). The CER formula is $C/(C + D) = 250/350 = 0.71$ or 71%.
   - The **EER** is the proportion of patients in the experimental group (those who received a crown) who experience the event (i.e., tooth loss). The EER formula is $A/(A + B) = 50/650 = 0.08$ or 8%.

2. **Relative risk (RR)** indicates likelihood that someone exposed to a risk factor (or treatment) will develop the disease (or experience a benefit) as compared with one who has not been exposed. This is expressed as the risk of the event in the exposed or experimental group (**EER**) $[A/(A + B)]$ divided by the risk of the event in the unexposed group, **CER** $[C/(C + D)]$ or EER/CER. A RR of >1 means a person is estimated to be at an increased risk (or benefit), whereas an RR of <1 means the person may be at decreased risk (or benefit). A RR = 1 means there is no apparent effect on risk or benefit at all.
   - Using the hypothetical example, the risk of an event (tooth loss) in the exposed group (those who received a crown) is 0.08 and the risk of an event (tooth loss) in the unexposed group is 0.71. The RR is calculated as EER/CER = $8/71 = 0.1126$, or 11.3%. That is, the RR of tooth loss is 11% for those who have received a crown.

3. **Absolute risk reduction (ARR)**, or **risk difference**, is the *absolute arithmetic difference* in the event rates between two groups (e.g., the control group [CER] and the experimental group [EER]). The formula for its calculation is $[C/(C + D)] - [A/(A + B)]$ or CER – EER. Substituting the numbers and values calculated, the ARR equals $0.71 - 0.8 = 0.63$ or 63%. The measure in this case indicates the percentage of people who are spared the adverse outcome (tooth loss) as a result of being exposed (i.e., receiving a crown).

4. **Relative risk reduction (RRR)** is *an estimate of the proportion of baseline risk* that is removed as a result of the therapy. It is calculated as the ARR between the treatment and control groups divided by the absolute risk among patients in the control group or (CER – EER)/CER. The easiest way to derive this value is by subtracting the RR (11.3%) from 1. In our example, the RRR is equal to 88.7%, which means that having a crown placed reduced the RR of tooth loss by 88.7% compared with that occurring among those in the control group (e.g., those who did not receive a crown).

5. **Odds ratio (OR)** is the proportion of patients with the target event divided by the proportion without the event, which yields the odds ratio of: $[A/B]/[C/D]$ or AD/BC or 3.3. This means that the odds of losing a tooth are more than three times greater for those who do not receive a crown than for those who do receive a crown after endodontic treatment. An OR = 1 indicates the effects of the treatment are no different than those of the control treatment. An OR >1 indicates the effects of the treatment are better than the effects of the control treatment and the opposite is true when the OR is <1.
   - The OR and RR do not indicate the magnitude of the absolute risk because they do not reflect the baseline risk. An RR of 50%, such as that discussed under Absolute and Relative Differences, may mean the treatment reduces the risk of an adverse outcome from 6% to 3% or from 80% to 40%, each of

TABLE 8-3

Statistics Used to Report Outcomes of Tooth Loss 5 Years[3,5–7]

Control event rate (CER): c/c+d Risk of tooth loss when not having a crown placed— control group	$250/350 = 0.71$ or 71%
Experimental event rate (EER): a/a+b Risk of tooth loss when having a crown placed—experimental group	$50/650 = 0.08$ or 8%
Absolute risk reduction (ARR): CER − EER Absolute arithmetic difference in the event rate between two groups	$0.71−0.08 = 0.63$ or 63%
Relative risk (RR): EER/CER Likelihood that someone exposed to a risk factor will develop the disease as compared to one who has not been exposed.	$.08/.71 = 0.113$ or 11.3%
Relative risk reduction (RRR): 1 − RR Estimate of the proportion of baseline risk that is removed as a result of the therapy.	$1−0.113 = 0.887$ or 88.7%
Odds ratio (OR): (A/B)/(C/D) Proportion of patients with the target event divided by the proportion without the event, which yields the odds ratio	$(50/600)/(250/100) =$ $0.083/2.5 = 0.33$ or 3.3
Numbers needed to treat (NNT): 1/AAR Reports the number of patients that need to be treated with the experimental treatment or intervention to achieve one additional patient who has a favorable response.	$1/0.63 = 1.59$, or 2 patients

which have very different clinical implications for deciding whether to use a treatment or not.

6. **Numbers needed to treat (NNT)** report the number of patients (teeth, surfaces, periodontal pockets) that need to be treated with the experimental treatment or intervention to have one additional patient (tooth, surface, periodontal pocket) benefit or to prevent one adverse outcome. NNT is calculated as 100/absolute difference (control rate − experimental rate), which is equal to 1/ARR. In the endodontic case, 1/ARR is (1/.63 = 1.59) equal to two patients. Therefore, only two patients would need a crown placed to have one additional patient benefit. The smaller the NNT is, the more effective the treatment. Thus, NNT and ARR represent the absolute arithmetic difference and take baseline risk into account, whereas results reported as relative risk or odds ratios do not.[3,5]

Table 8-3 summarizes the statistics that can be used to report outcomes using the hypothetical example presented in Table 8-2 of tooth loss 5 years after endodontic treatment comparing when a crown has been placed or not.

Understanding the measures of association and their differences are important because they can influence how outcomes are presented to patients and how clin-

ical decisions are made. Even though the information may be correct, presenting outcomes using relative findings rather than absolute differences tend to inflate the size of the effect and can influence a patient to accept the treatment a clinician may want the patient to select. Moreover, investigators have found that clinicians judge a therapy to be less effective when the results are presented in absolute terms[6,8] and that patients also are more likely to select a treatment when described in relative terms of RRR rather than its equivalent ARR or NNT.[9,10]

REPORTING OUTCOMES FOR SCREENING AND DIAGNOSTIC TESTS

Measures Used to Report Outcomes from Studies Related to Diagnosis

Diagnostic studies use measures other than those discussed so far. Screening and diagnostic tests need to have a high degree of accuracy in identifying the presence or absence of disease. It is important to note, however, that there is a distinction between the objectives of a screening test and a diagnostic test.[8] The objective of a screening test is to categorize individuals who are asymptomatic as being at high or low risk of a particular

TABLE 8-4

2 × 2 Contingency Table Related to Diagnostic Tests

Diagnostic Test Result	Disease Positive	Disease Negative
Test positive +	a (true positive)	b (false positive)
Test negative −	c (false negative)	d (true negative)
Totals	a + c	b + d

disease or condition, and not to make a definitive diagnosis. Further diagnostic procedures are then required for those who screen positive to determine their true status. In contrast, the objective of a diagnostic test is to establish an actual diagnosis and is often based on the presence of signs or symptoms of a condition or disease.[11]

The most commonly used measures of the relative validity of screening and diagnostic tests are sensitivity and specificity, as introduced in Chapter 4. Sensitivity and specificity answer the question: *What is the probability of getting a true test result given the patient has, or does not have, the disease/condition of interest?*

A 2 × 2 contingency table (Table 8-4) also can be used to define these terms related to diagnostic tests and illustrate how each is calculated.[3,6]

Sensitivity is the proportion of *people with a disease* or condition who *have a positive test* and is calculated using the formula a/(a + c). Ideally, all those with the disease/condition will have a positive test result, and all those who do not have the disease/condition will not have a positive test result. Under ideal conditions, the sensitivity of the test will be 100%; however, this is very rare. Conversely, a test with low sensitivity will *fail to detect disease/condition* in many of those who actually have it, thus yielding in a *false-negative* result.

Specificity is the proportion of *people free of a disease* who *have a negative test*, and can be determined using the formula d/(b + d). Again, the perfect test will

find that all those free of disease will have a negative test result, and those who have disease will not have a negative test result. Under these conditions, the specificity of the test will be 100%, yet this is extremely rare. Conversely, a test with low specificity will *falsely indicate disease* in many of those who do not have it, thus yielding in a *false-positive* result.

Tests must have both high sensitivity and specificity to be useful. For example, a new oral cancer screening test used on 500 people reports the results as seen in Table 8-5.

Using these findings, the sensitivity (a/a + c) is equal to 23/25 = 98% and the specificity (d/b + d) is equal to 460/475 = 97%. What this tells us is if a person has oral cancer, the probability that he has a positive result from using the new oral cancer screening test is 98%. Also, if a person does not have oral cancer, the probability that he has a negative result from the new test is 97%.

To calculate sensitivity and specificity it is presumed that the true disease status is known. However, when it is not known, which is often the case, then the probability of the test to give the correct result must be determined to make a correct diagnosis. The question now being answered is: *What is the probability that the patient actually has the disease given that the test results are known?*[8] To answer this question, the PPV and NPV for the test are calculated.[12]

The **positive predictive value (PPV)** is the proportion of people with a positive test who actually have

TABLE 8-5

Results of a New Oral Cancer Screening Test

	Disease Positive	Disease Negative
Test positive +	23 a (true positive)	15 b (false positive)
Test negative −	2 c (false negative)	460 d (true negative)
Totals	25 (a + c)	475 (b + d)

TABLE 8-6

Positive Predictive Values for New Oral Cancer Screening Test

	Disease Positive	Disease Negative	Totals
Test positive +	23 a (true positive)	15 b (false positive)	38 (a + b)
Test negative−	2 c (false negative)	460 d (true negative)	462 (c + d)
Totals	25 (a + c)	475 (b + d)	500

the target disorder = a/(a + b) or true positives/(true positives + true negatives). In other words, those who have the disease are correctly diagnosed as having it. Conversely, the **negative predictive value (NPV)** is the proportion of people with a negative test who do not have the target disorder = d/(c + d) (see Table 8-6).

In the oral cancer example, the PPV of the test on this group of people was therefore 23/38 = 0.605 = 61%. In other words, if someone in this group had a positive test, it was 61% likely that they had oral cancer. Conversely, the NPV was 460/462 = 0.996 = 99.6%, so that if someone in this group had a negative test, it was 99.6% likely that they did not have oral cancer.

PPVs and NPVs for a test vary according to the underlying prevalence of the disease or condition of interest in the group of people on whom it is applied.[8] For example, if a disease has a high prevalence in the population, positive test results are more likely to be correct, thus the positive predictive value will be relatively high. The reverse also is true. If a disease has a low prevalence, negative test results are more likely to be correct, and the negative predictive value will be relatively high.[8]

Other diagnosis and screening measures are **likelihood ratios**, both positive and negative. These are defined as the likelihood of a given test result in a patient with the disorder compared with the likelihood of the same result in a patient without the disorder. A positive likelihood ratio (+LR) is calculated as sensitivity/(1 − specificity) or [a/(a + c)] ÷ 1 − [b/(b + d)]; whereas a negative likelihood ratio (−LR) is calculated as (1 − sensitivity)/specificity or 1 − [a/(a + c)] ÷ d/(b + d).[5] The stronger +LR, the stronger the evidence for the presence or absence of disease. Likelihood ratio values above 5 are thought to be clinically useful[3] and those above 10 are considered strong evidence to rule in a diagnosis of a disease, whereas those below 0.1 are strong evidence to rule out the diagnosis of disease.[5] Again, inserting the values from the new oral cancer screen test results, the +LR would be equal to sensitivity (0.98) ÷ (1 − 0.97 = 0.3) or 98% ÷ 3% = 32.6. This means that a positive test result is 32.6 times more likely (strong evidence) to

have come from a person with the condition or disease (oral cancer) than from a person without the condition or disease. The results in calculating the −LR, (1 − sensitivity) ÷ specificity would be (1 − 0.98) ÷ 0.97 = 0.02, which means that a person with a negative test has a 1 in 50 chance of having oral cancer and provides us with strong evidence to rule out the diagnosis of disease.

REPORTING OUTCOMES FOR THE PROGRESSION OF TREATED DISEASE

Measures Used to Report Outcomes from Studies Related to Prognosis

For prognosis studies (i.e., the progression of treated disease), there are no specific calculations or statistics as there are with the other categories of studies.[3] Prognosis of diseases is based on having a representative sample of patients diagnosed at the early onset of their disease who are followed forward in time (inception cohort study design). Another key factor in providing a prognosis is follow-up of *at least 80%* of the cohort until the occurrence of a major study event or the end of the study.

Prognosis studies look at outcomes over time, such as the risk of an event occurring (e.g., the risk of a second heart attack for those who survived the first one). In the case of cardiovascular disease, control or treatment of certain risks, such as smoking, high cholesterol levels, high blood pressure, and diabetes could lower the risk of a second heart attack. When randomized controlled trials (RCTs) can be used to test specific treatments, they can provide reliable prognosis information, such as survival rates and disease progression data for both the treatment and placebo groups. Also, as previously discussed for treatment/prevention studies, the CER, EER, RRR, ARR, and NNT can be calculated to determine the number of events that can be prevented over a period of time (Table 8-7).[1,3]

Several resources are available that provide a further explanation of each measure, their relationship to

TABLE 8–7

Determining If the Results Are Important and Applicable to Your Patient[3,5]

	Are the Results Important?	*Are Results Applicable?*
Therapy/ prevention	Determine: Control event rate Experimental event rate Relative risk reduction Absolute risk reduction Numbers needed to treat	1. Is our patient similar to those in the study so that the results can be applied? 2. Is the treatment feasible in our setting? 3. What are our patient's potential benefits and harms from the therapy? 4. What are our patient's values and expectations for the outcome we are trying to prevent and the treatment offered?
Diagnosis	Determine: Sensitivity, specificity, and likelihood ratio Positive predictive value Negative predictive value	1. Is the diagnostic test available, affordable, accurate, and precise in our setting? 2. Will the resulting posttest probabilities affect our management and help our patient?
Prognosis	1. How likely are the outcomes over time? 2. How precise are the prognostic estimates? • Was there follow-up of at least 80% of the patient until the occurrence of either a major study end point or end of the study? • Were objective outcome criteria applied in a "blind" fashion?	1. Were the study patients similar to our own? 2. Will this evidence make a clinically important impact on our conclusions about what to offer or tell our patient?
Harm/etiology	In a randomized controlled trial or cohort study, determine relative risk In a case control study, determine relative odds Calculate the NNH (harm) or any odds ratio	Should valid, potentially important results change the treatment of our patient? 1. Is our patient similar to those included in the study so that the results apply? 2. What are the patient's risks of the adverse event and potential benefit from the therapy? 3. What are our patient's preferences, concerns, and expectations from this treatment? 4. What alternative treatments are available?

one another, and when to use each.[1,3,5,7] Detailed examples can be found in these references with McKibbon[3] and by Sackett[5] presenting clinically useful measures related to type of study: therapy/prevention, diagnosis, etiology, and prognosis. In addition, Needleman and Moles discuss issues specifically related to diagnostic studies and diagnostic outcome measures in *A Guide to Decision Making in Evidence-Based Diagnostics.*[8] Also, terms used to report outcomes are defined in the glossary section of this guidebook.

STATISTICAL VERSUS CLINICAL SIGNIFICANCE

Statistical significance refers to the likelihood that the results were unlikely to have occurred by chance at a specified probability level and that the differences would still exist each time the experiment was repeated. Therefore statistical significance is reported as the probability related to chance, or *p* value. Levels of statistical significance are set at thresholds at the point where the null hypothesis (the statement of no difference between groups) will be rejected, such as at $p < 0.05$ (where the probability is <5 in 100, or 1 in 20 that the difference occurred by chance), $p < 0.01$ (<1 in 100), or $p < 0.001$ (or <1 in 1,000).

Another concept related to statistical significance is the **confidence interval (CI)**, which quantifies the precision or uncertainty of study results. It usually is reported as 95% CI, which is the range of values within which we can be 95% sure that the true value for the whole population lies.[5] For example, in a comparison study of two sealant placement techniques, the mean difference in sealant loss in the two groups was 8 with a 95% CI of ± 2 sealants. This means that if the study was repeated

100 times, the mean difference would be between 6 and 10 sealants for 95% of the trials (8 ± 2).[5]

Statistical significance does not determine the practical or clinical implications of the data. For example, a difference of 0.05 to 1.0 mm in levels of attachment may be statistically significant; however, this small a difference could be due to measurement error or chance. Or, if there is no difference between two treatments (i.e., no statistically significant difference), then the investigation could be determining that a new treatment was as effective as the gold standard treatment.

Statistical significance is an important tool for determining the validity of a study's results; however, a number of techniques can increase the likelihood of obtaining statistically significant results. For example, as a sample size increases, the group differences needed to reach the *p* value decreases. Therefore any difference between treatment groups can become statistically significant if the studies are conducted with large enough sample sizes; however, this does not mean they are clinically important. Also, decreasing the variability within groups is another technique that will increase the likelihood that the differences between groups will be significant.[13] Thus, statistically significant results can be incomplete and provide misleading conclusions.[13]

Clinical significance is used to distinguish the importance and meaning of the results reported in a study and is not based on a comparison of numbers, as is statistical significance. It is possible for a study to have statistical significance without being clinically significant and vice versa. Statistical significance does not determine the practical or clinical implications of the data. For example, a new periodontal treatment "x" may increase levels of attachment 0.05 to 1.0 mm more than the standard treatment "y," which may be statistically significant; however, this small of a difference may not be clinically important in terms of saving periodontally compromised teeth. Also, the new treatment "x" provided to obtain these results may not take into account any additional training, special materials or instruments, patient time, or money.

Hujoel discusses clinical significance in terms of tangible versus intangible benefits, defining tangible as "those treatment outcomes that reflect how a patient feels, functions or survives" (p. 32).[14] These benefits include those that can be identified by the patient, such as improving quality of life, preventing tooth loss, or eliminating a painful abscess. On the other hand, intangible benefits are imperceptible to the patient and include such changes in probing depths because of scaling or the size of a periapical radiolucency after root canal treatment. Also, intangible benefits do not neatly translate into tangible benefits; *therefore, a treatment that provides tangible benefits has a higher level of clinical significance than those for which only evidence of intangible*

benefits exist. Ideally, clinical significant treatment would have both tangible and intangible benefits.[14] Other criteria for assessing clinical significance are the size of the treatment effect and meta-analyses. Measures of effect size analyze the degree to which the variables examined in a study explain the outcome or account for overall variability. For treatments that achieve a dramatic and immediate effect, reliable evidence may result from observations on a small number of patients (e.g., the effectiveness of general anesthesia). For small treatment effects, very rigorously designed controlled trials are required. The more likely a benefit can be obtained, the greater the clinical significance of the treatment.[14]

Meta-analyses summarize studies that have addressed the same question and statistically combine the results from the studies. By synthesizing the results, they can either confirm or strengthen the findings from smaller studies or find that treatments may not be as effective as originally thought (review Chapter 3 for more information on meta-analyses). Odds ratios are often used to report results when data from several studies are combined because the **OR** is not dependent on whether the risk of an event occurring was determined.

To determine clinical significance, one must go beyond the statistics and use all aspects of the evidence-based decision-making process (i.e., the patient's preferences and values) and the clinical circumstances in combination with the clinician's experience and judgment. For example, determining clinical versus statistical significance for Gail can be extrapolated from the RCT appraised in Chapter 6 discussing *The efficacy of pilocarpine and bethanechol upon saliva production in cancer patients with hyposalivation following radiation therapy*.[15] Statistically significant resting saliva volumes were reported for both treatments; however, when reviewing the mean saliva production for each treatment for females with functional salivary glands, the increase for pilocarpine was 3 mg/5 minutes and the increase for bethanechol was 1.5 mg/5 minutes. These results may not be a clinically significant increase that would relieve Gail's dry mouth. Conversely, the lack of statistical significance did not appear to make a difference in subjects reporting an increase in saliva from both pilocarpine and bethanechol, suggesting that even minor increases in saliva may produce a clinical and quality of life benefit. Also, improved taste and swallowing was reported with bethanechol and there were no significant differences in reported adverse side effects from the use of either drug.

Some helpful questions to consider when determining clinical significance are outlined in Fig. 8-2, which is the second component of Part F of the EBDM Worksheet. Using EBDM, scientific evidence is only one component to the decision making process. Synthesizing all four components is key to deciding a course of action

EBDM Worksheet Part F
Skill 4. Applying the Results of the Appraisal, or Evidence, in Clinical Practice
Questions to Ask Before Applying Evidence to Practice

			Rationale
1. Are the study groups similar enough to apply to my patient?	Yes	No	
2. Is this available, affordable, and appropriate for the patient in this setting?	Yes	No	
3. Will this help the patient meet his/her goals or address their chief complaint?	Yes	No	
4. Is the difference large enough to warrant the treatment?	Yes	No	
5. Adverse effects?	Yes	No	

Summary of scientific evidence:	Summary of your experience/judgment:	Summary of patient preferences/values:	Summary of clinical/patient circumstances:

Overall recommendations to the patient based on the EBDM process:

FIGURE 8–2 EBDM Worksheet Part F: Questions to Ask Before Applying Evidence to Practice.

EBDM Worksheet Part F
Skill 4. Applying the Results of the Appraisal, or Evidence, in Clinical Practice
Questions to Ask Before Applying Evidence to Practice

			Rationale
1. Are the study groups similar enough to apply to my patient?	(Yes)	No	Patients all experiencing hyposalivation
2. Is this available, affordable, and appropriate for the patient in this setting?	(Yes)	No	Rx items; ~$150/month without insurance
3. Will this help the patient meet his/her goals or address their chief complaint?	(Yes)	No	Nothing has helped Gail thus far; significant subjective benefits reported
4. Is the difference large enough to warrant the treatment?	(Yes)	No	Based on difference as reported by subjects in the study vs. statistical difference
5. Adverse effects?	(Yes)	No	Only minor effects were reported

Summary of scientific evidence:	Summary of your experience/judgment:	Summary of patient preferences/values:	Summary of clinical/patient circumstances:
Randomized cross-over study design; statistical significant (SS) findings for whole resting saliva but not stimulated saliva; SS improvement in subjective report of mouth wetness for both medications with increased percentage of those first receiving bethanechol (B); SS improvement in discomfort and taste with B and not pilocarpine.	Clinical significance appears to be more important in that subjects experienced reported saliva production/wetness improving their quality of life	Gail is seeking something to provide relief for her constantly dry mouth	Gail is on many medications that cannot be changed and are causing her dry mouth

Overall recommendations to the patient based on the EBDM process:
Based on the statistically significant report of patients experiencing an increase in saliva production or increased wetness, and only minor side effects, I would prescribe bethanechol to relieve Gail of her constant dry mouth.

FIGURE 8–3 Completed EBDM Worksheet Part F for Gail Case Scenario.

for your patient and is the third component of Part F of the EBDM Worksheet also included in Figure 8-2.

APPLYING THE EVIDENCE TO GAIL

The first section of Part F of the EBDM worksheet that asks for a summary of the outcome measures reported in the evidence could not be completed for Gail. The individual RCTs that were found related to Gail did not report results such as RRR, ARR, OR, and NNT. Keep in mind that the reporting of these outcome measures is just becoming more prevalent in the literature. Also, many of the RCTs were conducted in phases with multiple sets of data that were not clearly explained in the tables, thus making extrapolation of numerical data difficult. However, we can complete the following questions related to Gail in Fig. 8-3 (which is the second and third components of Part F of the EBDM Worksheet) based on the data available along with using our experience and judgment, the clinical/patient circumstances, and patient preferences and values. The following information is based on the study by Gorsky et al., on the efficacy of pilocarpine and bethanechol following radiation therapy.[15]

The answers to the above questions are yes, so it is time to discuss the related evidence with the patient. Based on the statistically significant report of patients experiencing an increase in saliva production or increased wetness, and only minor side effects, I would prescribe bethanechol to relieve Gail of her constant dry mouth. Also, bethanechol provided greater relief in terms of oral discomfort and taste. Pilocarpine and bethanechol cost approximately $150 per month without insurance and are appropriate for Gail to use in conjunction with her current medication regime. It will be up to Gail to determine if the price of the medication is affordable. After applying the evidence in practice, it is helpful to follow-up with patients to determine whether the recommendation was effective.

CONCLUSION

Understanding how statistical findings are presented can be difficult, especially because these may not have been part of a clinician's formal education. As with learning new knowledge and skills, these require time and practice. Although one may not be called on to perform calculations, knowing the difference between each of the statistics and when each is appropriate to use is key to translating research findings into practice to make informed patient care decisions.

REFERENCES

1. Evidence-based Medicine Working Group. *Users' Guides to the Medical Literature, A Manual for EB Clinical Practice.* Chicago: AMA Press, 2002.
2. Gigerenzer G, Edwards A. Simple tools for understanding risks: from innumeracy to insight. *BMJ.* 2003;327:741–744.
3. McKibbon A, Eady A, Marks S. *PDQ, Evidence-Based Principles and Practice.* Hamilton, Ontario: B.C. Decker Inc., 1999.
4. Centre for Evidence-Based Medicine. Glossary of terms in evidence-based medicine. Centre for Evidence-Based Medicine Web site. www.cebm.net/glossary.asp. Accessed April 8, 2007.
5. Sackett D, Straus S, Richardson W. *Evidence-Based Medicine: How to Practice & Teach EBM.* 2nd ed. London, England: Churchill Livingstone, 2000.
6. Centre for Evidence-Based Medicine. Critical appraisal. Centre for Evidence-Based Medicine Web site. www.cebm.net/critical_appraisal.asp. Accessed April 8, 2007.
7. Jaeschke R, Guyatt G, Shannon H, et al. Basic statistics for clinicians: 3. Assessing the effects of treatment: measures of association. *Can Med Assoc.* 1995;152:351–357.
8. Needleman I, Moles D. A guide to decision making in evidence-based diagnostics. *Periodontology. 2000* 2005;39:164–177.
9. Moher D. CONSORT Website News. CONSORT Web site. www.consort-statement.org/News/news.html. Accessed April 8, 2007.
10. Stroup D, Berlin J, Morton S, et al. Meta-analysis of observational studies in epidemiology, a proposal for reporting. *JAMA.* 2000;283:2008–2012.
11. Pereira-Maxwell F. *A-Z of Medical Statistics.* New York: Oxford University Press, 1998.
12. Altman D, Bland J. Diagnostic tests 2: predictive values. *BMJ.* 1994;309:102.
13. Glaros A. Statistical and clinical significance: alternative methods for understanding the importance of research findings. *J Irish Dent Assoc.* 2004;50:128–131.
14. Hujoel P. Levels of clinical significance. *J Evid Base Dent Pract.* 2004;4:32–36.
15. Gorsky M, Epstein J, Parry J, et al. The efficacy of pilocarpine and bethanechol upon saliva production in cancer patients with hyposalivation following radiation therapy. *Oral Surg Oral Med Oral Pathol Oral Radiol Endod.* 2004;97:190–195.

SUGGESTED ACTIVITIES

At this time, complete the quiz. Next, answer the critical thinking questions. Then complete Exercise 8-1, which asks you to complete Part F of the EBDM Worksheet for each of the 5 patient case scenarios.

QUIZ

Use Table 8-1 to answer questions 1 through 8. Match the appropriate formula to the correct statistical term.

1. _____	Event rate	a. AD/BC
2. _____	Experimental event rate (EER)	b. C/(C + D)
3. _____	Control event rate (CER)	c. (A + C)/N
4. _____	Odds ratio (OR)	d. A/(A + B)
5. _____	Absolute risk reduction (ARR)	e. EER/CER
6. _____	Relative risk (RR)	f. CER − EER
7. _____	Relative risk reduction (RRR)	g. 1/ARR
8. _____	Numbers needed to treat (NNT)	h. 1 − RR

Using this hypothetical example data for children that received sealants and developed caries, match the following terms to the correct number.

	Caries		
Sealants Placed	Yes	No	Total
Yes	86	416	502
No	474	24	498
Total	560	440	1,000

9. _____	Event rate	a. 0.17, or 17%
10. _____	Experimental event rate (EER)	b. 0.56, or 56%
11. _____	Absolute risk reduction (ARR)	c. 0.82, or 82%
12. _____	Relative risk reduction (RRR)	d. 0.78, or 78%

13. _____	Control event rate (CER)	a. 0.18, or 18%
14. _____	Relative risk (RR)	b. 0.95, or 95%
15. _____	Odds ratio (OR)	c. 1.28
16. _____	Numbers needed to treat (NNT)	d. 0.01

17. _____	Sensitivity	a. the proportion of people with disease or a condition who have a positive test
18. _____	Specificity	b. the likelihood of a given test result in a patient with the disorder compared with the likelihood of the same result in a patient without the disorder
19. _____	Positive predictive value (PPV)	c. the proportion of people free of a disease who have a negative test
20. _____	Likelihood ratio	d. the proportion of people with a positive test who actually have the target disorder

21. _____	Absolute risk reduction (ARR)	a. $a/(a + b)$
22. _____	Relative risk (RR)	b. $a/(a + c)$
23. _____	Relative risk reduction (RRR)	c. $[a/(a + c)] \div 1 - [b/(b + d)]$
24. _____	Numbers needed to treat (NNT)	d. $d/(b + d)$

25. The likelihood that the results were unlikely to have occurred by chance and that the differences would still exist if the experiment was repeated over and over.
    a. Clinical significance
    b. Statistical significance
    c. Likelihood ratio
    d. p value

CRITICAL THINKING QUESTIONS

1. Explain when a clinician might choose to present findings in relative terms versus absolute terms.

2. Discuss why predictive values are more useful than specificity and sensitivity in making a correct diagnosis.

3. Identify situations when clinical significance will outweigh statistical significance and vice versa.

EXERCISE 8-1

Complete Part F of the EBDM Worksheet for each of the five case scenarios. Use the RR, RRR, ARR, OR, LR, NNT, sensitivity, specificity, and predictive values. Then answer the application questions and summarize the scientific evidence, your experience/judgment, the patient preferences/values, and the clinical/patient circumstances, and finalize your overall recommendations for each of the five patient case scenarios. Again, use the studies that were identified and selected in Exercise 5-1 for each case to aid in this process.

Morty

Mr. Morty Kramer, a 55-year-old man, has been using unwaxed floss his whole life and flosses frequently. At his last dental appointment, he was treated by a new hygienist, who told him that he needed to change to using a waxed floss because it is more effective in removing plaque. Morty is happy with his current oral hygiene regimen and asks if he really needs to change.

Trevor

Trevor is a 27-year-old bartender who has used chewing tobacco for 13 years. He is a frequent user who chews almost 5 hours a day. He has just learned from his oral health care provider that he has developed precancerous lesions in the vestibular area where he holds the tobacco plug. This new information has motivated him to quit. Trevor knows he cannot quit by willpower alone because he has tried in the past. He wants to know if a non-nicotine aid in tobacco cessation is helpful in this endeavor, or if a nicotine patch is better in helping users permanently quit. He would like to know if behavioral therapy/counseling might help.

Dr. Bailer

Dr. Bailer recently graduated from dental school and is building a new dental practice. As he designs his building, he is trying to decide whether to purchase digital radiograph equipment or to use traditional radiography. He is interested in knowing the most accurate method for caries detection.

Jennifer

Your morning patient, Mrs. Jennifer Morris, comes to you distressed because of an article she read on the Internet about the dangers of mercury in her amalgam restorations. She is worried that her seven amalgam fillings are poisoning her. She is very concerned not only for her own health, but for her two young daughters that also have amalgam restorations. Jennifer doesn't want to replace her fillings if it isn't necessary, but needs proof that she and her children are going to be healthy.

To reassure your patient, you give her advice based on your clinical experience and judgment; however, she still seems very upset and troubled. You inform her that you will do a thorough search of the current scientific literature and get back to her with your findings. She seems more relaxed with this thought and leaves eager to hear from you soon.

Sam

Sam is a 49-year-old man with moderate periodontitis, who was recently diagnosed with type 2 diabetes mellitus. Sam's glycosylated hemoglobin (HbA1) is 12%, which places him in the category of poorly controlled diabetes. Sam is worried that his diabetes will increase his chance of losing his teeth. He wants to know the effect and impact diabetes now has on his oral health.

Outcome Measures for Five Patient Case Scenarios

Statistical Term	Morty	Trevor	Dr. Bailer	Jennifer	Sam
Control event rate (CER): c/c+d The proportion of patients in the control group (those who did not receive treatment), who experience the event.					
Experimental event rate (EER): a/a+b The proportion of patients in the experimental group (those who received a crown), who experience the event (i.e., tooth loss). The EER formula is A/(A+B).					
Absolute risk reduction (ARR): CER − EER Absolute arithmetic difference in the event rate between two groups					
Relative risk (RR): EER/CER Likelihood that someone exposed to a risk factor will develop the disease as compared to one who has not been exposed.					
Relative risk reduction (RRR): 1-RR Estimate of the proportion of baseline risk that is removed as a result of the therapy.					
Odds ratio (OR): (A/B)/(C/D) Proportion of patients with the target event divided by the proportion without the event, which yields the odds ratio.					
Numbers needed to treat (NNT): 1/AAR Reports the number of patients that need to be treated with the experimental treatment or intervention to achieve one additional patient who has a favorable response.					
Sensitivity: a/(a+c) The proportion of people with the disease or condition who have a positive test.					
Specificity: d/(b+d) The proportion of people free of disease who have a negative test.					
Positive predictive value (+PV): a/(a+b) The proportion of people with a positive test who actually have the target disorder.					
Negative predictive value (-PV): d/(c+d) The proportion of people with a negative test who do not have the target disorder.					

EBDM Worksheet Part F
Questions to Ask Before Applying Evidence to Practice
Skill 4. Applying the Results of the Appraisal, or Evidence, in Clinical Practice

			Rationale
1. Are the study groups similar enough to apply to my patient?	Yes	No	
2. Is this available, affordable, and appropriate for the patient in this setting?	Yes	No	
3. Will this help the patient meet his/her goals or address their chief complaint?	Yes	No	
4. Is the difference large enough to warrant the treatment?	Yes	No	
5. Adverse effects?	Yes	No	

Summary of scientific evidence:	Summary of your experience/judgment:	Summary of patient preferences/values:	Summary of clinical/patient circumstances:

Overall recommendations to the patient based on the EBDM process:

Please fill this page out for each case scenario

CHAPTER 9

Evaluating the Process and Your Performance

SKILL 5

Evaluating the Process and Your Performance.

PURPOSE

The final step in evidence-based decision making (EBDM) is evaluation of the effectiveness of the process. Mastering the skills of EBDM takes practice and reflection and a clinician who is new to the steps should not be discouraged by early difficulties encountered. Evaluating the process of EBDM may include a range of activities such as examining outcomes related to the health/function of the patient or patient satisfaction. Self-evaluation of developing skills is a most critical aspect in mastery of EBDM. With an understanding of how to effectively use EBDM, you can quickly and conveniently stay current with scientific findings on topics that are important to you and your patients.

OBJECTIVES

After completing this chapter, readers will be able to:

1. Rate your ability to perform the various aspects of EBDM:
   - Formulate a searchable question.
   - Identify sources and levels of evidence.
   - Use the PICO question to search for and find evidence.
   - Critically appraise the evidence that you find.
   - Apply the results to patient care.
2. Based on the results of your self-evaluation, identify additional learning needs and strategies that fit with your learning styles and preferences.
3. Develop a plan to incorporate EBDM into your clinical practice on an ongoing basis.

SUGGESTED ACTIVITIES

Quiz
Critical Thinking Questions
Exercise 9-1

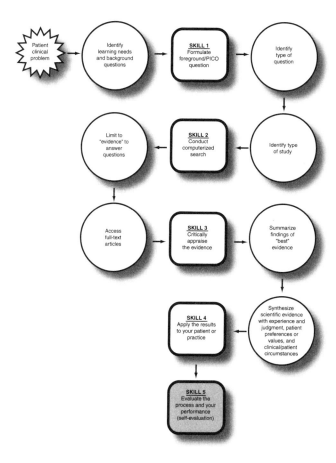

EVALUATION OF THE EBDM PROCESS

Ultimately, effective implementation of EBDM will enhance patient care by allowing the busy clinician to manage the challenge of the ever-increasing body of scientific evidence.[1] EBDM, practiced on a consistent basis, will foster a system of health care that takes into account clinical judgment, patient values, and the most current scientific evidence. Studies have shown that courses in EBDM can convey the theoretical principles, but, if not practiced on a consistent basis, skill development will lag.[2] The ability to accurately reflect on performance and modify behavior to improve outcomes is a hallmark of expertise.[3] Expertise in EBDM begins with evaluating each of the steps of the EBDM process.

A crucial first step in developing the skills of EBDM is recognizing the need to ask questions. Clinicians make countless decisions each day. Every decision will not require the development of a PICO question, but some patient situations will provide the opportunity to use EBDM. Statements made by colleagues, in the media, or by company representatives may also offer the opportunity to implement the EBDM process by asking an answerable question. If you are finding opportunities to pose answerable clinical questions, you are beginning to develop the skills of an EBDM practitioner. Next, reflecting on each step of the process of EBDM is necessary to build your skills. There are several guides available to help practitioners evaluate their EBDM skills.[4,5]

EVALUATION TOOLS

The University of Sheffield's School of Health and Related Research Section on Information Resources[5] identifies four targeted questions that an EBDM practitioner can use to evaluate performance:

- Were my questions answerable?
- Did I find good evidence quickly and efficiently?
- Did I appraise the evidence effectively?
- Did my integration of the appraisal with my own expertise and the unique features of the situation lead to a rational, acceptable management strategy?

A more in-depth framework for this evaluative process, the EBDM Evaluation Tool or Part G of the EBDM Worksheet is presented in Exercise 9-1 at the end of this chapter. The EBDM Evaluation Tool breaks the process of EBDM into the five skills needed to apply the EBDM process introduced in Chapter 1.

First, converting information needs/problems into clinical questions so that they can be answered, which asks one to develop a question with four parts: patient, intervention, comparison, and outcomes along with alternative keywords that can be used in searching. **SECOND**, based on the question, one should consider the most *appropriate study types and the levels of evidence* that will be needed to answer the question confidently. **THIRD**, Conducting a computerized search with maximum efficiency for finding the best external evidence with which to answer the question. **FOURTH**, Critically appraising the evidence for its validity and usefulness (clinical applicability) after articles are identified. **FINAL**, Applying the results of the appraisal, or evidence, in clinical practice.

As discussed earlier, EBDM is not finding evidence and blindly applying the evidence to patient care. EBDM requires the integration of the best available evidence with clinical judgment and patient's unique needs, values, and preferences. Evaluating the process and your performance is the final skill in the process of becoming skilled in EBDM.

THE CONTINUUM OF COMPETENCE

The EBDM Evaluation Tool is based on the continuum of competence that has gained acceptance in professional education.[3] The continuum begins at *novice*, proceeds through stages of *beginner, competent, proficient,* and culminates in *expert* (Fig. 9-1). Students in professional education enter at the novice stage and through a series of learning experiences progress toward the development of expertise. The dental educational curriculum must demonstrate that graduates have developed competence, leaving the development of proficiency and expertise for later.[6] Expertise develops over time with practice experiences and reflection. The developmental stages of competence can also be applied to the development of EBDM skills. The first stage in the road to competence is *beginner*. At this level of the learning curve, students can understand theory but cannot always connect it to practice. The second tier on the continuum is *competent*. Students here can integrate theory with practice and demonstrate the basic abilities of EBDM. *Proficient* practitioners can combine analytical thinking with intuitive experience with greater depth and breadth of understanding in a wide range of cases. The final phase of competence is *expert*, which involves effortlessly completing the EBDM process as normal, easily incorporating each aspect into everyday practice while blending the highest level of judgment and skills. Table 9-1 compares the behaviors of a beginner-novice, a competent practitioner, and a practitioner who is proficient moving to expertise in problem solving situations analogous to using EBDM.

The learning curve for many aspects of EBDM is quite steep. However, with time and practice, the climb toward becoming an expert evidence-based practitioner is easily within reach. Identifying learning needs based on the self-evaluation tool can aid in improving performance of the EBDM process. Reviewing the related sections of this workbook can strengthen the weak areas. Additional tutorials and resources are available on the Web site www.usc.edu/ebnet, which has valuable resources related to each aspect of the EBDM process.

DEVELOPING AN EVIDENCE-BASED DATABASE AND LIBRARY

Organizing the results of the EBDM process eliminates duplication of efforts, documents methods used to

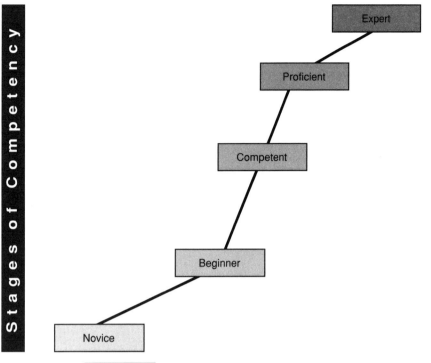

FIGURE 9–1 The continuum of competence.

TABLE 9–1

Behaviors During Problem Solving

Novice	Beginner	Competent	Proficient	Expert
Slow	Hesitant	Analytical and deliberate	Greater breadth and depth of understanding	Fast and fluid
Requires lecture and labs to learn theory and rules	Requires practice in multiple applications with varying situations	Demonstrates basic abilities of a safe, independent practitioner	Demonstrates abilities with a wide range of situations	Uses intuition and experience without conscious analytic thinking
Lacks understanding	Understands theory, but cannot always connect it to clinical situations	Integrates theory and practice. Has a variety of possible solutions to problems	Provides leadership even when situation is ambiguous and outcome is uncertain	Effortlessly completes tasks as normal
Requires frequent guidance and evaluation	Rule bound; tries to implement textbook approaches	Ability to discern pertinent information	Adapts to circumstances; not locked into any one particular strategy	Blends highest level of judgment and skill
Externally motivated	"Trial-and-error" efforts to solve the problem using one approach at a time	Able to independently implement a course of action	Settles on the "best course of action" after quick review of options, but willing to change course if results are not satisfactory	Is able to combine all decision-making skills to solve a problem with little effort

Adapted from Hendrickson et al.[3]

Evidence-Based Dentistry Rx

Name: _____   Date: _____

Question: _____

Search Strategy: _____

_____

_____

Number of valid studies: _____

Results of studies _____

_____

_____

_____

_____

Recommendations: _____

_____

_____

_____

_____

Supervisor's signature _____

FIGURE 9–2   Evidence-based dentistry prescription (adapted from Werb and Matear).[2]

develop evidence, and enables practitioners to have evidence at their fingertips. Sites such as the Cochrane Library (www.cochrane.org) and the Centre for Reviews and Dissemination of York University (www.york.ac.uk/inst/crd/) offer databases of topics that have been critically appraised using evidence-based methods. These sites provide quick access to high-quality information that is updated on a regular basis to assure current information.

The practitioner committed to providing evidence-based health care may also want to create a personal evidence-based database or library of topics that they have developed through an evidence-based process. Werb and Matear suggested an educational form, the EBD Rx, that can be developed when an evidence based review is collected.[2] The EBD Rx is presented in Fig. 9-2.

For more detailed documentation of the results of EBDM, the EBDM worksheet Parts A–F presented in this book can be included in a personal library of EBDM

results or as an evidence-based portfolio. These documents cover each of the skills necessary for using EBDM and include the PICO question, the search strategy including levels of evidence, selected abstracts, selected literature, critical appraisal, and the recommendation to the patient based on the evidence and three other aspects of EBDM. A brief summary of the intervention/treatment provided or decision made, the outcome, and any future considerations could also be included if appropriate. Patient name, chart number, and other relevant demographic information would aid in subsequent retrieval and organization. Through this documentation, you can update evidence as it becomes available, identify major influences in decision making, and track different aspects of care and their related outcomes.

In an educational setting, integration of EBDM into course requirements can be accomplished by a faculty course director or by the faculty collectively as an outcomes database for the clinical program. For example, have students document patient problems, the PICO question investigated and the evidence found that either contributed to or influenced their clinical decision making. Begin this process as they enter clinic and have it continue throughout their education. Creating a database would allow faculty to monitor the development of a student's EBDM and critical thinking skills over time. Ultimately, implementation of EBDM in health care has the potential to foster translation of research findings into clinical practice, reduce variability of care provided, and improve patient health outcomes. Implementation of EBDM instruction and practice into the clinical setting has the greatest potential to achieve these improvements in patient outcomes.[1]

CONCLUSION

The final step in the EBDM process is evaluation of the process and your performance. The path for development of expertise in any skill involves learning the basic steps followed by practice in applying the skills; however, practice without reflection on how to improve is trial-and-error learning. The reflective practitioner is continually self-assessing results of their actions to enhance their abilities and development of expertise.

This is also the case with development of skills in EBDM. The practitioner who makes time to apply *and* evaluate the results of EBDM will develop expertise and foster optimal patient care.

REFERENCES

1. Coomarasamy A, Khan K. What is the evidence that postgraduate teaching in evidence based medicine changes anything? A systematic review. *BMJ.* 2004;329:1017–1022.
2. Werb S, Matear DW. Implementing evidence-based practice in undergraduate teaching clinics: a systematic review and recommendations. *J Dent Educ.* 2004;68:995–1003.
3. Hendricson WD, Andrieu SC, Chadwick G, et al. Educational strategies associated with development of problem-solving, critical thinking, and self-directed learning. *J Dent Educ.* 2006;70: 925–936.
4. Sackett D, Richardson W, Rosenberg W, et al. *Evidence-Based Medicine: How to Practice and Teach EBM.* New York: Churchill Livingstone, 1997.
5. University of Sheffield School of Health and Related Research Section on Information Resources. Evidence based health care process, Section 7: Evaluate your performance. www.shef.ac.uk/scharr/ir/mschi/unit2/7evaluate.htm. Accessed September, 30, 2006.
6. American Dental Association Commission on Dental Accreditation. *Accreditation standards for dental education programs.* ADA, Chicago, IL 2002.

SUGGESTED ACTIVITIES

At this time, complete the quiz. Next, answer the critical thinking questions. Then complete Part G of the EBDM worksheet. Finally, outline a plan for implementing EBDM into your practice.

QUIZ

1. The first step in development of expertise in EBDM is:
   a. recognizing the need to ask questions.
   b. learning to critically appraise evidence.
   c. framing searchable questions.
   d. applying evidence to patient care.

2. Four broad questions can be used to evaluate performance in EBDM. They do NOT include
   a. Are my questions answerable?
   b. Was my search reasonably fast and efficient?
   c. Did my search produce full text articles?
   d. Was I able to evaluate the quality of the evidence I found?

3. The final step in development of expertise in EBDM is
   a. recognizing the need to ask questions.
   b. conducting a search for evidence.
   c. applying the evidence to patient care.
   d. evaluating your own developing abilities in the EBDM process.

4. A practitioner who is able to effortlessly complete the EBDM process can be characterized as
   a. a beginner.
   b. a novice.
   c. competent.
   d. an expert.

5. Overall, I would rate my current skill level in EBDM as
   a. beginner.
   b. novice.
   c. competent.
   d. proficient.
   e. expert.

6. The final step in evidence-based decision making is
   a. recognizing the need for PICO.
   b. conducting a computerized search.
   c. critically appraising the search results.
   d. applying results to practice.
   e. evaluation of the process and your performance.

7. EBDM is effective for you as a practitioner if the results
   a. are geared toward patient preferences and values.
   b. are obtained efficiently.
   c. help improve the patient outcomes.
   d. All of the above.

CRITICAL THINKING QUESTIONS

1. Discuss the biggest barriers you face in implementing EBDM. What measures can you take to overcome those barriers?

_____

_____

_____

_____

_____

_____

_____

_____

_____

2. Now that you have completed the EBDM process, discuss how you can use these skills to provide better care for your patients.

_____

_____

_____

_____

_____

_____

_____

_____

_____

3. Now that the process is complete for all of the cases, discuss how you could have improved one of the five evidence-based skills to obtain better results for Morty, Trevor, Jennifer, Dr. Bailer, or Sam.

_____

_____

_____

_____

_____

_____

_____

_____

_____

NOTES

EXERCISE 9-1

Evaluate your EBDM skills using Part G of the EBDM Worksheet. Rate your performance of each aspect of EBDM by identifying where you are on the competence continuum. Outline how you plan to strengthen your weaknesses in the Comments section.

Name_____Topic_____

EBDM Worksheet Part G

Skill 5. Evaluating the Process and Your Performance

Rate your performance of each aspect of EBDM by identifying where you are on the Competence Continuum based on the definition of each. Outline how you plan to strengthen your weaknesses in the comments section.

Novice	Beginner	Competent	Proficient	Expert
Lacks full understanding, requires frequent guidance and needs to learn theory and rules	Understands the theory but cannot always connect it to practice	Integrates theory and practice and demonstrates the basic abilities of EBDM	Mixes analytical thinking with intuitive experience with greater depth and breath of understanding in a wide range of cases	Effortlessly completes tasks as normal, blending the highest level of judgment and skill

Skill 1. Converting Information Needs/Problems into Clinical Questions so That They Can be Answered

1. PICO, Asking Good Questions

Rate your level of ability to:

	Novice	Beginner	Competent	Proficient	Expert
• Define the specific PICO components					
• Formulate a well-built question derived from a patient case using the PICO format					
• Identify additional keywords based on PICO					
• Use the PICO process for my own questions					
• Use the PICO process with staff, students, colleagues					
Comments:					

2. Research Design and Sources of Evidence and Levels of Evidence

Rate your level of ability to:

	Novice	Beginner	Competent	Proficient	Expert
• Distinguish between publication types					
• Identify and select appropriate study designs according to the type of question being asked					
• Define the levels of evidence					
Comments:					

Skill 2. Conducting a Computerized Search with Maximum Efficiency for Finding the Best External Evidence with Which to Answer the Question

3. Finding the Evidence: Using PICO to Guide the Search

Rate your level of ability to:

	Novice	Beginner	Competent	Proficient	Expert
• Identify inclusion criteria					
• Use PubMed to search the literature					
• Identify MeSH with the PubMed MeSH Database					
• Use MeSH terms when searching					
• Combine search terms with Boolean Operators					
• Limit the search based on inclusion criteria					
• Track the process with the Search History					
• Search different/multiple databases					
Comments:					

Name_____Topic_____

EBDM Worksheet Part G

Skill 5. Evaluating the Process and Your Performance (continued)

Skill 3. Critically Appraising the Evidence for Its Validity and Usefulness

4. Critical Appraisal of the Evidence
Rate your level of ability to:

	Novice	Beginner	Competent	Proficient	Expert
• Identify where the selected study is in the heirarchy of levels of evidence					
• Screen and select appropriate abstracts					
• Critically appraise the validity of research studies					
• Use evidence to answer a PICO question					
Comments:					

Skill 4. Applying the Results of the Appraisal, or Evidence, in Clinical Practice

5. Applying the Evidence to Practice
Rate your level of ability to:

	Novice	Beginner	Competent	Proficient	Expert
• Incorporate EBDM into practice					
• Present research findings to patient					
• Use the scientific evidence as a resource in clinical decision making					
Comments:					

Skill 5. Evaluating the Process and Your Performance

6. Self-Evaluation
Rate your level of ability to:

	Novice	Beginner	Competent	Proficient	Expert
• Conduct a self-evaluation					
• Make improvements based on past experiences					
• Identify additional learning needs					
Comments:					

Complete EBDM Worksheet

Name_____   Topic_____

EBDM Worksheet

PART A. *Skill 1. Convert Information Needs/Problems into Clinical Questions So That They Can Be Answered*

1. **Write your Background questions—general knowledge inquiries that ask the who, what, where, when, how, and why for what you need to learn more about.**

   1._____

   2._____

   3._____

   4._____

   5._____

   6._____

   7._____

   8._____

   9._____

   10._____

2. **Summarize the findings from your Background questions.**

   1._____

   2._____

   3._____

   4._____

   5._____

3. **Define your question using PICO by identifying: Problem, Intervention, Comparison Group, and Outcome.**

   Your question should be used to help establish your search strategy.

   Patient/Problem _____
   Intervention _____
   Comparison _____
   Outcome _____

4. **Write out your question.**

   _____

   _____

5. **Identify the type of question/problem appropriate for your patient. Circle one:**

   Therapy/Prevention   Diagnosis   Etiology, Causation, or Harm   Prognosis

PART B. *Understanding the Publication Type So That Appropriate Studies Can Be Identified*

1. Type of study (Publication Type) to include in the search: Check all that apply, and then number from highest (#1) to lowest level of evidence.

❑ _____Meta-Analysis	❑ _____Systematic Review	❑ _____Randomized Controlled Trial
❑ _____Clinical Trial	❑ _____Practice Guideline	❑ _____Review
❑ _____Cohort Study	❑ _____Case Control Study	❑ _____Case Series or Case Report
❑ _____Editorials, Letters, Opinions	❑ _____Animal Research	❑ _____In Vitro/Lab Research

PART C. *Skill 2. Conducting a Computerized Search with Maximum Efficiency for Finding the Best External Evidence with which to Answer the Question*

1. List main topics and alternate terms from your PICO question that can be used for your search. Circle MeSH Terms.

_____	_____
_____	_____
_____	_____
_____	_____
_____	_____
_____	_____

2. List your inclusion criteria—gender, age, year of publication, language, etc.

List irrelevant terms that you may want to exclude in your search.

3. List where you plan to search (i.e., EBM Reviews, MEDLINE, PubMed, CINAHL, Cochrane).

4. List the web addresses of the Internet search and attach the information summary.

WEBSITE ADDRESS	INFORMATION FOUND

5. Attach your search strategy here (printed from the PudMed History tab), or fill in the table.

	Search History	Results
#1		
#2		
#3		
#4		
#5		
#6		
#7		
#8		
#9		
#10		
#11		
#12		
#13		
#14		
#15		

PART D. *Skill 3. Critically Appraising the Evidence for Its Validity and Usefulness*

1. Summarize the results of the evidence that you found for your patient.

Article Reference #1:			
Type of Study:	**Level of Evidence:**	**Does this answer my question? YES NO**	**Will I use this for my patient? YES NO**
A. Are the results of the trial valid?			
B. What are the results?			
C. Will the results help my patients?			

Article Reference #2:			
Type of Study:	**Level of Evidence:**	**Does this answer my question? YES NO**	**Will I use this for my patient? YES NO**
A. Are the results of the trial valid?			
B. What are the results?			
C. Will the results help my patients?			

Article Reference #3:			
Type of Study:	**Level of Evidence:**	**Does this answer my question? YES NO**	**Will I use this for my patient? YES NO**
A. Are the results of the trial valid?			
B. What are the results?			
C. Will the results help my patients?			

Article Reference #4:			
Type of Study:	**Level of Evidence:**	**Does this answer my question? YES NO**	**Will I use this for my patient? YES NO**
A. Are the results of the trial valid?			
B. What are the results?			
C. Will the results help my patients?			

Article Reference #5:			
Type of Study:	**Level of Evidence:**	**Does this answer my question? YES NO**	**Will I use this for my patient? YES NO**
A. Are the results of the trial valid?			
B. What are the results?			
C. Will the results help my patients?			

PART E. Evaluating the Websites Where Information Pertinent to the Patient Is Found

Skill 3. Critically Appraising the Evidence for its Validity and Usefulness

	URL of page evaluated: http://	URL of Page evaluated: http://
Information about the Site		
Domain	❏ .com, .org, .net ❏ .edu ❏ .mil/.gov/ ❏ other:_____	❏ .com, .org, .net ❏ .edu ❏ .mil/.gov/ ❏ other:_____
Is the domain appropriate for the content?	❏ Yes　　❏ No	❏ Yes　　❏ No
Is the purpose and mission of the website appropriate for the information posted?	❏ Yes　　❏ No	❏ Yes　　❏ No
Ownership	❏ Private:_____ ❏ Public:_____	❏ Private:_____ ❏ Public:_____
Webmaster Contact Info	**Name:** **Address:** **Email:**	**Name:** **Address:** **Email:**
Date information was posted	**mm/dd/yr**	**mm/dd/yr**
Date site was last updated	**mm/dd/yr**	**mm/dd/yr**
Credibility of Information		
Is the information current?	❏ Yes　　❏ No	❏ Yes　　❏ No
Is it clear who wrote the page/information?	**Name:** **Email:** **Credentials:**	**Name:** **Email:** **Credentials:**
Is the writer qualified to discuss the topic?	❏ Yes　　❏ No	❏ Yes　　❏ No
Is there bias, opinions?	❏ Yes　　❏ No	❏ Yes　　❏ No
Is the information referenced, reliable, and accurate from print/published research?	❏ Yes　　❏ No **Desribe your answer:**	❏ Yes　　❏ No **Desribe your answer:**
Are the sources current and well-documented?	❏ Yes　　❏ No	❏ Yes　　❏ No
Are there links to more resources?	❏ Yes　　❏ No	❏ Yes　　❏ No
What is the purpose of the information? Check all that apply.	❏ Inform　❏ Explain ❏ Persuade　❏ Disclose ❏ Sell　　❏ Advertise	❏ Inform　❏ Explain ❏ Persuade　❏ Disclose ❏ Sell　　❏ Advertise
Sponsorship		
Is a sponsor clearly identified?	❏ Yes　　❏ No	❏ Yes　　❏ No
Is there an Advisory Board or are there consultants?	❏ Yes　　❏ No	❏ Yes　　❏ No
Are the partnerships or advertisements clear?	❏ Yes　　❏ No	❏ Yes　　❏ No
Is the information usable based on the above?	❏ Yes　　❏ No	❏ Yes　　❏ No

PART F. *Skill 4. Applying the Results of the Appraisal, or Evidence, in Clinical Practice*

1a. Outcomes Measures for Article #1

CER	EER	ARR	RR	RRR	OR	NNT	Sensitivity	Sensitivity	NPV	PPV

2a. Questions to ask prior to applying evidence to practice for Article #1   Rationale

1. Are the study groups similar enough to apply to the patient?	YES	NO	
2. Is this available, affordable, and appropriate for the patient in this setting?	YES	NO	
3. Will this help the patient meet his/her goals/address his/her chief complaint?	YES	NO	
4. Is the difference large enough to warrant the treatment?	YES	NO	
5. Are there adverse events that influence a potential recommendation?	YES	NO	

1b. Outcome Measures for Article #2

CER	EER	ARR	RR	RRR	OR	NNT	Sensitivity	Sensitivity	NPV	PPV

2b. Questions to ask prior to applying evidence to practice for Article #2   Rationale

1. Are the study groups similar enough to apply to the patient?	YES	NO	
2. Is this available, affordable, and appropriate for the patient in this setting?	YES	NO	
3. Will this help the patient meet his/her goals/address his/her chief complaint?	YES	NO	
4. Is the difference large enough to warrant the treatment?	YES	NO	
5. Are there adverse events that influence a potential recommendation?	YES	NO	

1c. Outcome Measures for Article #3

CER	EER	ARR	RR	RRR	OR	NNT	Sensitivity	Sensitivity	NPV	PPV

2c. Questions to ask prior to applying evidence to practice for Article #3   Rationale

1. Are the study groups similar enough to apply to the patient?	YES	NO	
2. Is this available, affordable, and appropriate for the patient in this setting?	YES	NO	
3. Will this help the patient meet his/her goals/address his/her chief complaint?	YES	NO	
4. Is the difference large enough to warrant the treatment?	YES	NO	
5. Are there adverse events that influence a potential recommendation?	YES	NO	

1d. Outcomes Measures for Article #4

CER	EER	ARR	RR	RRR	OR	NNT	Sensitivity	Sensitivity	NPV	PPV

2d. Questions to ask prior to applying evidence to practice for Article #4   Rationale

1. Are the study groups similar enough to apply to the patient?	YES	NO	
2. Is this available, affordable, and appropriate for the patient in this setting?	YES	NO	
3. Will this help the patient meet his/her goals/address his/her chief complaint?	YES	NO	
4. Is the difference large enough to warrant the treatment?	YES	NO	
5. Are there adverse events that influence a potential recommendation?	YES	NO	

1e. Outcome Measures for Article #5

CER	EER	ARR	RR	RRR	OR	NNT	Sensitivity	Specificity	NPV	PPV

2e. Questions to ask prior to applying evidence to practice for Article #5   Rationale

1. Are the study groups similar enough to apply to the patient?	YES	NO	
2. Is this available, affordable, and appropriate for the patient in this setting?	YES	NO	
3. Will this help the patient meet his/her goals/address his/her chief complaint?	YES	NO	
4. Is the difference large enough to warrant the treatment?	YES	NO	
5. Are there adverse events that influence a potential recommendation?	YES	NO	

3. Using evidence-based decision makeing, scientific evidence is only one component to the decision-making process. Please synthesize all four of the components to decide on a course of action for your patient.

Summary of Scientific Evidence:	Summary of your Experience/Judgment:	Summary of Patient Preferences/Values:	Summary of Clinical/Patient Circumstances:

Overall Recommendations to the Patient based on the EBDM Process:

PART G. *Skill 5. Evaluating the Process and Your Performance*

Rate your performance of each aspect of EBDM by identifying where you are on the competence continuum. Outline how you plan to strengthen your weaknesses in the comments section.

Novice	Beginner	Competent	Proficient	Expert
Lacks full understanding, requires frequent guidance, and needs to learn theory and rules	Understanding the theory but cannot always connect it to practice	Integrates theory and practice and demonstrates the basic abilities of EBDM	Mixes analytical thinking with intuitive experience with greater depth and breadth of understanding in a wide range of cases	Effortlessly completes tasks as normal, blending the highest level of judgment and skill

Skill 1. Converting Information Needs/Problems into Clinical Questions So That They Can Be Answered

1. PICO, Asking Good Questions

Rate your level of ability to:	Novice	Beginner	Competent	Proficient	Expert
• Define the specific PICO components					
• Formulate a well-built question derived from a patient case using the PICO format					
• Identify additional keywords based on PICO					
• Identify inclusion criteria					
• Use the PICO process for your own questions					
• Use the PICO process with staff, students, colleagues					

Comments:

2. Research Design and Sources of Evidence and Levels of Evidence

Rate your level of ability to:	Novice	Beginner	Competent	Proficient	Expert
• Distinguish between publication types					
• Identify and select appropriate study designs according to the type of question being asked					
• Define the levels of evidence					

Comments:

Skill 2. Conducting a Computerized Search with Maximum Efficiency for Finding the Best External Evidence with which to Answer the Question

3. Finding the Evidence: Using PICO to Guide the Search

Rate your level of ability to:	Novice	Beginner	Competent	Proficient	Expert
• Identify inclusion criteria					
• Use PubMed to search the literature					
• Identify MeSH with the PubMed MeSH Database					
• Use MeSH terms when searching					
• Combine search terms with Boolean Operators					
• Limit the search based on inclusion criteria					
• Track the process with the Search History					
• Search different/multiple databases					

Comments:

Skill 3. Critically Appraising the Evidence for Its Validity and Usefulness

4. Critical Appraisal of the Evidence

Rate your level of ability to:	Novice	Beginner	Competent	Proficient	Expert
• Identify where the selected study is in the hierarchy of levels of evidence					
• Screen and select appropriate abstracts					
• Critically appraise the validity of research studies					
• Use evidence to answer a PICO question					

Comments:

Skill 4. Applying the Results of the Appraisal, or Evidence, in Clinical Practice

5. Applying the Evidence to Practice

Rate your level of ability to:	Novice	Beginner	Competent	Proficient	Expert
• Incorporate EBDM into practice					
• Present research findings to patient					
• Use the scientific evidence as a resource in clinical decision making					

Comments:

Skill 5. Evaluating the Process and Your Performance

6. Self-Evaluation

Rate your level of ability to:	Novice	Beginner	Competent	Proficient	Expert
• Conduct a self-evaluation					
• Make improvements based on past experiences					
• Identify additional learning needs					

Comments:

GLOSSARY

Absolute Difference The arithmetic difference between rates.

Absolute Risk The absolute arithmetic difference in the event rates between two groups (e.g., the control group [CER] and the experimental group [EER]). The formula for its calculation is $[C/(C + D)] - [A/(A + B)]$ or CER − EER.

Article Reviews A one- to two-page structured abstract along with an expert commentary highlighting the most relevant and practical information of the study being reviewed.

Background Question General knowledge inquiry that asks who, what, where, when, how, or why.

Bias Systematic deviations from the underlying truth.

Boolean Operators Words used to associate terms in a PubMed/MEDLINE search that limit results of a search by allowing the combination of search terms or concepts. The three Boolean operators are AND, OR, and NOT.

Case Control Studies Studies that make observations about possible associations between the disease of interest (lung cancer) and one or more hypothesized risk factors (tobacco use). Case-control studies are retrospective in that subjects *already have a certain disease or condition* and are compared with a representative group of disease-free persons (controls) from the same population.

Case Reports A description of a single patient case report. These are observations and do not use a control group with which to compare outcomes.

Case Series Descriptions of a series of patients with a similar situation that report observations and do not use a control group with which to compare outcomes.

CINAHL The Cumulative Index to Nursing & Allied Health, an online database that provides access to journals related to nursing and other allied health fields, including dental hygiene.

Clinical Practice Guidelines Systematically developed statements to assist practitioner and patient decisions about appropriate health care for specific clinical circumstances.

Clinical Significance The importance and meaning of the results reported in a study related to tangible and intangible benefits.

Cohort Study A study that makes observations about the association between a particular exposure or a risk factor (e.g., tobacco use) and the subsequent development of a disease or condition (e.g., lung cancer). In these studies, subjects do not presently have the condition of interest (lung cancer) and are followed over time to see at what frequency they develop the disease/condition as compared with a control group that is not exposed to the risk factor (tobacco use) under investigation.

Confidence Interval (CI) Quantifies the precision or uncertainty of study results. It usually is reported as 95% CI, which is the range of values within which we can be 95% sure that the true value for the whole population lies.

Control Event Rate (CER) The proportion of patients in the control group (those who did not receive treatment), who experience the event (i.e., tooth loss). The CER formula is $C/(C + D)$.

Diagnosis Questions Questions that look for evidence to determine the degree to which a test is reliable and useful; the selection and interpretation of diagnostic methods or tests that establish the power of an intervention to differentiate between those with and without a target condition or disease.

Double-Blind Randomized Controlled Trials Double-blind trials contain the rigor and methodology of a randomized controlled trial, but in addition are conducted so that neither the patient nor the investigator knows whether the patient is receiving the experimental treatment or the control treatment.

Event Rate The proportion of patients in a group in whom the event is observed.

Evidence-Based Decision Making The formalized process and structure for using the skills for identifying, searching for, and interpreting the results of clinical research so that the best scientific evidence is considered in conjunction with experience and judgment, patient values, and clinical circumstances when making patient care decisions.

Evidence-Based Journals Journals that provide concise and easy-to-read summaries of original and review articles selected from the biomedical literature based on specific inclusion criteria.

Evidence-Based Medicine The integration of best research evidence with clinical expertise and patient values.

Experimental Event Rate (EER) The proportion of patients in the experimental group (those who received treatment), who experience the event (i.e., tooth loss). The EER formula is $A/(A + B)$.

Experimental Studies Studies in which the researcher controls or manipulates the variables under investigation, such as in testing the effectiveness of a treatment. These studies are the most complex and include randomized controlled trials and controlled clinical trials.

Foreground Question A specific question that is structured to find a precise answer and phrased to facilitate a computerized search. It should include four parts that identify the patient problem or population (P), intervention (I), comparison (C), and outcome(s) (O), referred to as PICO.

Gold Standard Test The test or measure considered the ultimate or ideal.

Gray Literature Newsletters, reports, working papers, theses, government documents, bulletins, fact sheets, conference proceedings, and other publications not controlled by commercial publishers.

Harm, Causation, Etiology Questions Questions used to identify causes of a disease or condition including iatrogenic forms and to determine relationships between risk factors, potentially harmful agents, and possible causes of a disease or condition.

Inception Cohort Studies Studies in which the cohort of subjects are all initially free of the outcome of interest and are followed until the occurrence of either a major study end point or end of the study.

Levels of Evidence Hierarchy of research study designs based on the rigor of the methodology used and its ability to minimize bias, allowing the user to put confidence in the results. Different hierarchies exist based on the type of questions asked, e.g., treatment vs. diagnosis or prognosis.

Likelihood Ratios The likelihood of a given test result in a patient with the disorder compared with the likelihood of the same result in a patient without the disorder. A positive likelihood ratio (+LR) is calculated as sensitivity/(1 – specificity) or $[a/(a + c)], 1 - [b/(b + d)]$; whereas a negative likelihood ratio (–LR) is calculated as (1 – sensitivity)/specificity or $1 - [a/(a + c)], d/(b + d)$.

Medical Subject Headings (MeSH) A controlled vocabulary of biomedical terms to index articles, catalog books, and other holdings, and to facilitate searching within MEDLINE.

MEDLINE The bibliographic database of the National Library of Medicine (NLM) that contains bibliographic citations and author abstracts that cover the fields of medicine, nursing, dentistry, and veterinary medicine.

Meta-Analysis The statistical process commonly used with systematic reviews that involves combining the data from multiple individual studies into one analysis.

Negative Predictive Value The proportion of people with a negative test who do not have the target disorder = $d/(c + d)$.

Nonexperimental studies Studies in which the researcher does not give a treatment, intervention, or provide an exposure (i.e., data are gathered without intervening to control variables). Examples of nonexperimental studies include cohort studies, case control studies, case series, and case reports.

Numbers Needed to Treat The number of patients (teeth, surfaces, periodontal pockets) that need to be treated with the experimental treatment or intervention to have one additional patient (tooth, surface, periodontal pocket) benefit, or to prevent one adverse outcome. NNT is calculated as 1/ARR.

Odds Ratio The proportion of patients with the target event divided by the proportion without the event, which yields the odds ratio of: [A/B] / [C/D] or AD/BC.

OVID An information search platform that includes Ovid Gateway and SilverPlatter and allows users to access electronic citations, including journals, books, and databases, with innovative tools to browse, search, retrieve, and analyze critical information.

PICO A systematic process for converting information needs/problems into a clinical question that defines the patient problem, intervention, comparison, and outcome. (See also Foreground Question)

Positive Predictive Value The proportion of people with a positive test who actually have the target disorder = a/(a + b) or true positives/(true positives + true negatives).

Primary Research   Original research publications that have not been filtered or synthesized and include individual RCTs, and well-designed nonrandomized control studies.

Prognosis Questions   Questions that depend on studies that estimate the clinical course or progression of a disease or condition over time and anticipate likely complications (and prevent them).

PubMed   An online database that provides free access to citations from biomedical literature, including MEDLINE, as well as access and links to other molecular biology resources.

Qualitative Research   Nonexperimental research that conducts studies in natural settings in an attempt to understand an event from the point of view of the participants. It seeks to provide depth of understanding and does so through answering questions such as what, how, and why. It explores issues in more depth with those experiencing the issue rather than testing a hypothesis to answer questions such as how many or what proportion. It uses an interpretive, naturalistic approach that focuses on how individuals or groups view and understand their surroundings and construct meaning out of their experiences.

Quantitative Research   Research that focuses on establishing cause-and-effect relationships through testing a specific hypothesis and reporting the results in statistical terms.

Randomized Controlled Trial (RCT)   Involves at least one test/experimental treatment or intervention and one control treatment that can be a placebo treatment or no treatment.

- Concurrent enrollment of subjects and follow-up of the experimental test- and control-treated groups,
- Assignment of subjects to either the experimental treatment/intervention group or the control/placebo group through a random process, such as the use of a random-numbers table, and
- Follow-up of both groups to determine the outcome.

Relative Difference   The proportion or percent increase or difference.

Relative Risk   Likelihood that someone exposed to a risk factor (or treatment) will develop the disease (or experience a benefit) as compared with one who has not been exposed. The formula is the risk of the event in the exposed or experimental group, **EER** [A/(A + B)] divided by the risk of the event in the unexposed group, **CER** [C/(C + D)] or EER/CER.

Relative Risk Reduction   An estimate of the proportion of baseline risk that is removed as a result of the therapy. It is calculated as the ARR between the treatment and control groups divided by the absolute risk among patients in the control group or (CER-EER/CER).

Scientific Evidence   The product of well-designed and well-controlled research investigations that minimize sources of bias, considered the synthesis of all valid research studies that answer a specific question. The body of knowledge that has been derived from multiple studies investigating the same phenomena.

Secondary Research   Filtered or synthesized publications of the primary research literature and include systematic reviews or meta-analyses.

Sensitivity   The proportion of *people with disease* or condition who *have a positive test* and is calculated using the formula a/(a + c).

Specificity   The proportion of *people free of a disease* who *have a negative test*, and can be determined using the formula d/(b + d).

Statistical Significance   The likelihood that the results were unlikely to have occurred by chance at a specified probability level and that the differences would still exist each time the experiment was repeated. Therefore, statistical significance is reported as the probability related to chance, or *p* level.

Systematic Reviews   Summary of two or more primary research studies that have investigated the same specific phenomenon or question. This scientific technique defines a specific question to be answered and uses explicit predefined criteria for retrieval of studies, assessment, and synthesis of evidence from individual RCTs and other well-controlled methods. Methods used in SRs parallel those of RCTs in that each step is thoroughly documented and reproducible.

Therapy/Prevention Questions   Questions that look for answers that determine the effect of treatments that avoid adverse events, improve function, and are worth the effort and cost.

Validity   The degree to which a study appropriately answers the question being asked or appropriately measures what it intends to measure.

INDEX

Note: Page numbers followed by f indicate figure; those followed by t indicate table.

NOTES

NOTES

NOTES

NOTES

NOTES